SELF-CARE
REFORM

HOW TO DISCOVER YOUR OWN PATH TO GOOD HEALTH

RUSTY GREGORY

MS, CSCS, CWC

PUBLICATION: DECEMBER, 2013
Copyright © 2013 Rusty Gregory

ISBN-13: 978-1494293826
ISBN-10: 149429382X

A TESTAMENT TO CHANGE:

"As a family physician for over 30 years, I have counseled, encouraged and supported hundreds of patients on their way to a lifestyle of better health and fitness. Unfortunately, even the "success stories" more often than not are either short lived or fall short of their intended long-term goals.

"In his book, *SELF-CARE REFORM: How to Discover Your Own Path to Good Health*, Rusty Gregory, personal trainer and certified wellness coach, offers a new methodology, and an exciting alternative to those more common approaches used today in promoting health and fitness that all too often result in discouragement and failure. His program changes the origin of the wellness vision and ensuing plan of action to come directly from the reader instead of a formula imposed by an outside source.

"Having been a client of Rusty Gregory and as a referring physician, friend and colleague of many of his clients and fellow trainers, I have witnessed the evolution of these successful methods and techniques. Allow me to share the reasons I wholeheartedly endorse and recommend his easy to read, practical and timely book.

"In the area of health and fitness, there are many applicable formulas for success, including those so called scientifically based or proven. Examples are those of the American Heart Association, the American Diabetic Association, etc. Despite decades of such studies and guidelines, relatively few individuals are able to make or sustain the behaviors that result in even relatively limited goals of weight, blood chemistry, or aerobic fitness improvements. The reason is that these programs are designed as 'one size fits all' and do not allow for the individual to reprogram behaviors for continued success. Mr. Gregory's methodology answers and corrects those shortcomings. He engages the reader with a unique series of questions at the end of each chapter. In responding to those questions, the reader: (1) identifies his/her individual needs and deficiencies in the areas of health, nutrition, fitness, etc.; (2) identifies causes and existing barriers of past failures to be overcome; (3) formulates reasonable and specific goals in each of the areas discussed; and (4) in achieving stepwise success with the individual goals, selects and begins practicing and building upon the maintenance of those behaviors. Journaling is another tool that assists the reader in maintaining lifestyle changes. Mr. Gregory supports the reader in participating in a more intimate, personal stepwise program that leads to very real and attainable success. It allows for change and growth with the individual's needs and life patterns in order to 'Discover' his/her own path to health.

"I would enthusiastically recommend Rusty Gregory's book to all my patients – those who are recovering and treating serious illness as well as those who want to reduce long term risk. It will be the best therapeutic and preventative medicine they can take."

Andrew H. Weary, M.D.

CONTENTS

FOREWORD i

INTRODUCTION 1

1. WHAT'S YOUR STORY? 5

2. ARE YOU ALIVE AND WELL?....................... 12

3. WHAT DOES IT MEAN TO BE WELL? 16

4. YOU: YOUR OWN WORST ENEMY? 21

5. CREATING A VISION & S.M.A.R.T. GOALS 35

6. UNDERSTANDING LIFELONG CHANGE 53

7. DEVELOPING A ROUTINE 75

8. CREATING AN ENVIRONMENTALLY-SAFE
   WELLNESS PROGRAM!.................................80

9. FROM THE INSIDE OUT 89

10. THE ZONE VS. DISRUPTION 132

11. CARPE DIEM 136

12. FREQUENTLY ASKED QUESTIONS............... 143

13. STRATEGIES FOR GETTING STARTED 148

BENEFITS AND SUGGESTIONS.....................155

ACKNOWLEDGMENTS.....................................166

ABOUT THE AUTHOR.....................................167

ENDNOTES...169

FOREWORD

Throughout *SELF-CARE REFORM: How to Discover Your Own Path to Good Health*, I use the words health and wellness interchangeably. More often than not, these words are associated with the absence of disease, injury, and pain. As a result, we seek treatment only when we are sick and hurting. This leads to the faulty belief that everything is okay if we are not sick or hurting, and if we are, just pop a pill or take a shot. There are appropriate times and places for medication, but we have become all too quick to opt for the fastest or easiest remedy, not necessarily the healthiest. Health and wellness encompass all of this and so much more. Health and wellness also include living the best life possible. Optimal health and wellness include reaching the peak levels of our emotional, physical, mental, and spiritual being. When we reach the highest levels in these areas, we are truly alive and well.

There is a risk of injury with exercise. Therefore, always consult a physician before starting any exercise program and a registered dietician or nutritionist before starting any nutrition program. This book is not meant to diagnose mental, physical, emotional, or spiritual illnesses. Nor is it meant to prescribe medications or treatments for any such conditions. Although I believe everyone can learn something about his or her relationship with wellness from this book, individual circumstances may require professional counseling and/or medical treatment.

INTRODUCTION

Health care costs are spinning out of control, with many Americans unable to afford monthly health insurance premiums. More and more money is spent on the diagnosis and treatment at the doctor's office and preventative care is relatively ignored. So, what is behind these increasing prices? First, the government subsidizes big agriculture that produces wheat and corn for the masses. This drives the cost of food down making it cheap to eat regardless of the illnesses these grains cause. At the other end, small organic farmers are squeezed out because of the high cost of doing business. Second, there is an increase in the number of people with preventable chronic diseases. Because of the health complications associated with eating wheat, corn, other grains, and sugar the health care industry spends billions of dollars on cancer, heart disease, type 2 diabetes, Alzheimer's and obesity. Too few people are eating healthy, exercising regularly, plus soaring stress levels, have created a society that is often slow to start or to sustain a healthy way of living. The need for self-care programs is imperative.

What are we to do as a country to solve this problem? The answer: act individually! *If you take care of yourself, health care will take care of itself.* Yes, this means we must all do our part, not only for ourselves, but for the greater good as well. The state of health care in America is in crisis. Costs are going up and quality health care is in danger of going down. Self-care reduces illness and therefore reduces personal insurance claims. This is a simplistic approach to an issue we have made complicated. By taking charge of our health through eating healthy, exercising regularly, managing our weight and stress levels, and balancing our life and work schedules, we can make a significant difference in the cost of our health care.

It's up to YOU, America!

SELF-CARE REFORM: How to Discover Your Own Path to Good Health asks questions designed to generate purposeful reflection on your own wholeness. It also provides tools that lead you to life-giving and health-promoting behaviors. We often need such tools to start and to maintain a wellness program. Using these tools helps you re-frame your behaviors in order to meet your needs for well-being.

When it comes to motivation or trying to establish new routines and habits, we have all experienced the difficulty of change. I answer the question "What makes us do the things we do (regarding our wellness), even though we know we shouldn't do them?" to bring a deeper understanding to your thought processes. This deeper awareness will help prepare you to change and to move away from destructive behaviors.

This book is for everyone who wants to improve health and fitness in any wellness area, from work/life balance to stress management to creating an exercise routine. There is a twelve-week wellness/gratitude journal as a supplement to this book to help motivate and assist you in charting your progress in all areas of wellness. The journal is also your blueprint for personally designing a healthy future that is specific to your individual wants and needs.

In this book, I will help you develop a greater understanding of how body awareness, motivation, confidence, strengths, opportunities, and dreams can affect your effort towards a wellness plan. By learning what is realistic for you, and what you want and need, you are better able to design a program that will work best for you. This self-designed lifestyle will be based solely on your wants and needs. This is why already de-signed programs labeled "scientifically based" or "proven" do not often work long-term: they have not been created by the person who is to live out this new lifestyle.

I use practical experience and theoretical knowledge to connect with my readers. Your level of readiness, willingness, and commitment combined with your emotional state all contribute to your level of motivation. This book is full of anecdotes to help stir those emotions inside of you and get you to act. I want you to see that all of the changes my clients have made can happen to you, too. I have accumulated over twenty years of client stories, and a variety of coaching techniques, to help motivate and inspire anyone who wants to start and sustain a self-care program. To protect individual identities all the names in my stories have been changed. An in-depth look at the change process, a mindful approach, and designing your own wellness vision and S.M.A.R.T. goals in detail and with accountability will equip you with the tools for success.

This book doesn't take the place of psychological therapy. If you find that dealing with the past and how it is manifested in you today needs to be addressed before you can begin a self-care program, then it is wise to consider professional therapy.

SELF-CARE REFORM: How to Discover Your Own Path to Good Health combines the unique experiences of a personal fitness trainer; the academic knowledge gained from a master's degree in kinesiology; the certifications of a wellness coach, strength and conditioning specialist, and cancer exercise specialist; and the contributions of an expert in health and fitness for dailyRx.com.

CHAPTER 1
WHAT'S YOUR STORY?

The most overlooked issue in the health, fitness, and wellness industry is starting and sustaining a self-care program.

With New Year's Day quickly approaching, you find yourself mulling over what areas of your life most need your attention. As you assess last year's resolution to lose those thirty unwanted pounds, an overwhelming sense of defeat dominates your thinking. *If only last year my father-in-law had not had a prolonged illness culminating in his death; if we hadn't had such a brutally cold winter, and my daughter had not sustained a concussion that kept her out of school for six weeks, then I could have accomplished my goal.*

Does this scenario sound familiar? Or, do you lose interest in an exercise plan that seemed so important just weeks before? Do the results you expect not equal the effort you are putting forward? Unfortunately, these are just a few of the ways in which a well-intentioned health-promoting goal goes astray.

After three years of dipping his toe into the weight-loss waters, Michael, one of my personal training clients, told me it was time for him to jump in completely. It was time for the weight to come off. He had reached rock bottom. So, over the next eleven months, he dropped a staggering 200 pounds by increasing his aerobic exercise, maintaining his weight room workouts, and drastically changing his diet. I tell you Michael's story to get you to focus on YOUR story. Maybe you need a comeback, or maybe you just need to maintain what you are doing; whatever it is, I hope you will pay attention to what is happening now with your health and wellness.

At some point, most people temporarily commit to a healthier way of living. I see it every day: we start an exercise program, promise our spouses to work less and be home with the family more, vow to push away second, third, and fourth helpings at mealtime, and swear that this is the year to quit smoking. More appropriately, we should be asking, "What is going to keep me motivated?" Anyone can be moved to action when all eyes are on her and desperation is all-consuming. We can become highly motivated when recovering from a heart attack or receiving a cancer diagnosis. What is there to keep the drive alive? Our new commitments tend to lose energy and fade in importance over time. What then?

Michael's story is awe-inspiring, even if it had ended right there. But it didn't, and over the past four years he gained back half his lost weight. How could someone with a newfound look, energy, and confidence fall back into the very routines that got him in trouble in the first place? Ironically, Michael is one of the most motivated people I know. Due to injuries he sustained earlier in life, he finds himself unable to work out when pain, his old friend, revisits him. He begins to eat and drink, and the cycle starts all over again. As most of us know, it is not uncommon to lose weight only to regain it, over and over again. So, what's the answer?

How are we to better our lives through weight loss/management, health, fitness, nutrition, and work/life balance, when time, stress, and energy are not on our side? This is exactly what happened to Michael; he crossed what he thought was the finish line only to realize, later, it was just the starting line. Had Michael implemented tools that would work best for *him* once he reached his weight-loss goal, his success would have continued.

Arthur, my ninety-six-year-old personal training client, and his wife, Margaret, age 89, exemplify how incorporating certain tools and techniques can make the difference between life and death. As a result of connecting what they value—mobility and general health—to their daily lifestyle of weight training and aerobic exercise, they strengthened their commitment to their cause. Few workouts end without Arthur thanking me for helping him extend and enrich his life.

We are a nation fixated on fat, body weight, quick fixes, and how these relate to beauty. When you add that together, you get: "I want to lose weight so that I will look great in my bathing suit, NOW!" If we reach that point of "beauty," often we then do whatever it takes to stay there, including crazy diets, dehydration, unhealthy exercise habits, and, in some cases, drugs. You can probably see where this ends up. Unfortunately, this scenario totally dismisses the importance of self-care. Instead, by making wellness a lifestyle, we reap the health benefits of practicing life-giving health-promoting behaviors, including looking better—beauty becomes the byproduct, not the focal point of our efforts.

The fitness industry is fraught with the "most intense" fat loss workouts, the "latest and greatest" fitness equipment, and the "most effective" diets for weight loss. The wheel gets reinvented, over and over again. Over the last twenty years or so, fitness centers and gyms have offered ridiculously low monthly dues to entice people to join. By doing so, they over-book their memberships, knowing that only a small percentage of members will actually show up to use their facilities. *Sell, sell, sell* is the fitness industry's mantra! All of this sensationalism is marketed as if it were the be-all and end-all, when in fact it is merely pushing a product or service on a desperate and gullible consumer.

What those in the fitness industry who market the latest and greatest fitness equipment or exercise program don't want you to know is, all you need to do is *overload* the system you seek to enhance in order to reap the benefits of exercise. By overloading, I mean safely stressing a system of the body. If you stress the cardiovascular system, for example, by increasing your heart rate to a target zone for twenty to thirty minutes, then your cardiovascular system comes back stronger than it was before because of the body's ability to adapt. The same is true for all other forms of exercise.

The most overlooked issue in the health, fitness, and wellness industry is starting and sustaining a self-care program. In the following chapters, I address this very important issue by providing you with tools to assist you in engaging in and maintaining lifelong health-promoting behaviors.

We live in a society where tips, advice, and other recommendations are a dime a dozen. It seems that everywhere we go we are told what to do. Although advice can be given effectively at certain times, at other times it creates resistance—an opposition that only pushes us farther away from the desired behavior. This is not a book about how to exercise, what to eat, or what stress management techniques work best. This book will lead you to discover YOUR OWN path to wellness.

For years I have sought the answer to the questions "What makes each one of us feel alive? What will it take to help someone reach that 'alive' place?" I decided to write this book after exploring these questions on a weekly health, fitness, and wellness blog for the previous two-and-a-half years. I also wanted to include my Christian "walk" as the foundation of my wellness journey. I have discovered that writing a book about maximizing your health and wellness without considering your relationship with your Creator is like writing a book about light and not mentioning fire or electricity. It can't be done adequately. My hope is that you will realize what makes you feel alive in your physical and spiritual realms, as well as emotionally and mentally, and *seek* it out.

As a personal trainer and wellness coach, I wear many hats. I have been called on to serve as a trainer, coach, counselor, network and resource guide, sounding board for business ideas, relationship "expert," friend, and confidant. However, none of these seems to be more important than serving as a question-asker. The more quality questions I ask, the more discoveries my clients make about their health. When discoveries are made, pathways and possibilities are generated, leading toward a healthier way of living. We all share the universal need for well-being and face similar obstacles in meeting that need. By regularly practicing self-care, we better our lives, the lives around us, and the world at large.

For those who think they are well because they are thin, think again. There is so much more to health, fitness, and wellness than dress size or what the scale says. Actually, I train several people who are overweight but are much more fit than the average non-fit, thin person. Therein lies the deception. We ALL need exercise, proper dietary intake and hydration, to manage our stress, adequate amounts of sleep, to manage our weight, to balance work and family, and to implement other health practices to live life to its fullest.

You see what people really want when you look at what they are willing to sacrifice in order to get it. People seek to meet their needs in the best ways they know how. Unfortunately, those ways often lead to higher stress levels, an unhealthy diet, inactivity . . . you get the picture. Consequently, health problems such as heart disease, diabetes, hypertension, and obesity follow. So what's the answer? How can we reverse this trend plaguing our country?

1 First, identify what is most important to you right now. What do you value? Would you like to run a marathon in six months or establish a healthy lifestyle to generate energy well into your elderly years? Whatever it is, name it so you can move to the next step.

2 Second, gather as much information as you can about this new endeavor you plan to tackle. How realistic is this behavior? Is it cost-prohibitive? What challenges might you encounter along the way? What is your "Plan B"?

Third, develop a plan of action. Once you have put into practice your new plan, DON'T LOOK BACK! Follow your routine. You will find that those things that were difficult before you began your routine are less difficult now.

Lifelong change does not by itself support a sense of willpower, or temporary motivation, which is a constant battle. Having the ability to resist temptation at a given moment does not necessarily bring about lasting change. That is why short-term diets do not work. They are a temporary fix for a permanent need (well-being). They do not address lasting change—that challenges your ability to make the right decision regardless of your circumstances. Well-being must become a lifestyle.

Let's get started!

Questions from page 9

Answers here:

1. What is most important to you right now? Sleep; Lowering ✓ (10-15) Cholesterol; dropping 10 lbs; Having time to enjoy what I like most. Hanging out w/ friends (Can't do that COVID19) (same sex!

What do I value — Relaxing friendships, health; Marriage Get rid of my perfectionist/ procrastination mode. Learn to manage time to remember stuff you need/want to a

CHAPTER QUESTIONS:

1. What has derailed you from your past New Year's resolutions or promises to yourself?

   I lose focus, forget, get distracted, cravings rule; no one to make me accountable. ⚹WEATHER ⚹ PROCRASTINATION

2. What is your main reason for reading this book? Are you looking for a comeback, wanting to seriously address your health for the first time, or searching for ways to sustain your current self-care program?

   definetly ways to sustain a better self-care program

3. List the areas of wellness that you would like to address right now (exercise, weight loss, nutrition, stress management, work/life balance), in the order of their importance to you.

   exercise — add more frequency & intensity
   weight 10-15 !
   Time management.
   Add some spiritual routines & relationships

CHAPTER 2
ARE YOU ALIVE AND WELL?

Nothing has more influence on your behavior than your emotional state.

Recently, my eleven-year-old son David told me he had asked one of his classmates to be his Valentine. When I was in the fifth grade, I would ask a girl to "go with me." If she said "yes," then I had a girlfriend with whom I seldom, if ever, talked. If she said "no," I would try to survive the humiliation of rejection. My son's crush said "yes." Our family was so proud. My oldest daughter, Brittany, took David to the store to buy a Valentine's Day gift. They returned with a stuffed teddy bear, a bag of Hershey Kisses, and a decorative gift bag. Less than twenty-four hours later, David had eaten half of her gift: the chocolate. When I asked him why he did this, he said, *"There was more than she could eat."* Although a bit twisted and misguided there, David would tell you that eating chocolate makes him feel alive, to a point.

What do you know about what makes you feel most alive—that something that evokes the deepest emotions inside you? Is it spending time with family and friends, or viewing a sunset at the ocean or in the mountains? A profound spiritual experience? Or, completing a day of high-energy foods and a fantastic workout?

Many of us set the cruise control and navigate through life on autopilot. And why not? Isn't life a lot easier and less stressful when we don't pay attention to the mundane details that pop up every day? I suppose so, but how will you become your best if you're sitting on the sidelines and not experiencing all that life has to offer?

By discovering what makes you feel alive, especially in the area of your wellness, you can practice those activities that stir your emotions and push you to act on energy-giving behaviors. Nothing has more influence on your behavior than your emotional state. Positive emotions tend to promote positive behaviors and negative emotions tend to generate negative behaviors.

Fifty-three-year-old Bill exemplifies this very point. He is morbidly obese and carries around a great deal of negative emotional baggage. His emotional state always dictates the energy of his workouts. When Bill shows up late for his scheduled appointment, he is dragging and sluggish. He's quiet, pensive, and very slow in all he does. It's like pulling teeth to get him to do anything of significance in the gym. These times totally drain me; it's a real effort just to get through the hour because I often feed off the energy of my clients. When Bill's positive emotional tank is full, he is much more lively and energetic and is more engaging during the workout. He moves from exercise to exercise much faster, and as a result I almost bounce around the gym. I estimate that he does close to twice as much work when he is "feeling good." The same is true with his workouts outside the gym and his dietary habits. Bill reports sedentary living and poor dietary intake when he's "down," and a more active lifestyle and better food choices when he's "up."

I try to evoke the positive in Bill when he's struggling. I ask, "What's the best thing that's happened to you in the past week?" Or "What are three things that made you smile this week?" These questions are a good starting point to redirect his emotional swing. Focusing on those things that I know bring him joy and excitement is another technique. He usually lights up like a Christmas tree when I ask him about his daughter or his New York Giants football team. By diverting his attention away from the negativity on which he is focused, the negative energy drains away and loses momentum. At this point, an energy shift occurs. New vigor and enthusiasm takes root, and positive emotions start to flourish. Consequently, Bill's workouts often go from sluggish to energetic.

CHAPTER QUESTIONS:

1. If you had no obligations for a day, what life-giving activities would you perform?

Play in the garden; Shop for plants? I'd love to _and steps_ plan a meditative nature trail in my back yard w/ a water feature. Get together w/ a friend for lunch or dinner

2. What can you do to pull yourself out of a negative emotional slump?

Listen to music, Dance, go for a walk. take a long shower make some art? which I rare rarely do.

3. What strengths of yours can you draw upon when you are sluggish emotionally during your workouts? (?)

Listen to more of my choice of music. [Start a collection for my workouts.] My sense of humor. Remember what I'm grateful for

CHAPTER 3
WHAT DOES IT MEAN TO BE WELL?

What makes us do the things we do, even though we know we shouldn't do them?

The question "What makes us do the things we do (regarding our wellness), even though we know we shouldn't do them?" has perplexed me my entire professional life. Many of us choose destructive behaviors, such as a poor diet, sedentary lifestyle, smoking, and non-monitored stress. Why? We are bombarded by ads offering ways to live a better, more fulfilling life through performing self-care. But still we choose the "easier" and "more comfortable" life that is familiar.

Every day I address this question and how it relates to each one of my clients. My four conclusions as to why we stay with the familiar rather than change for the better are:

1. Our identity becomes so wrapped up in our illness that we wouldn't know who we were if we made a change for the better.

Consider John 5:1–9. Jesus had gone to a Jewish festival in Jerusalem. In the city there was a pool where many disabled people gathered. One man in particular had been immobilized for thirty-eight years. Jesus saw the man lying there and was told he had been ill for quite some time. Jesus asked the man if he wanted to get well. The man responded by telling him there was no one to help him into the water and that others would always go ahead of him. It was at this time that Jesus healed the man, telling him to get up and walk.

The very nature of asking someone if they want to get well implies that not all people want to do what it takes to change and get better. At first glance, it seems absolutely ludicrous to think someone would rather be unhealthy than choose do to the things necessary to be well. However, the overwhelming and daunting task that becoming someone different conjures up can paralyze a person to the point of inaction.

Sixty-four-year-old William believed that the change process was too difficult. Even though a regular aerobic exercise program and a change in his diet would improve his blood pressure, cholesterol levels, and add life to his years, he felt making that change would require too much of him. Many of his friends lived a similar lifestyle: little physical activity, a reckless diet, and plenty of alcohol. He once told me, "If I make these changes that you suggest, I wouldn't have any friends; these activities are what we do when we get together."

---

2. **Some get comfortable with their illness, and it's easier to stay where they are because otherwise they would have to become responsible and accountable for normal day-to-day living.**

When we enable those who choose not to change and be well, we perpetuate the no-change cycle. This cycle creates a mindset of not having to be responsible and accountable for what we choose to do. In turn, this mind-set leads to an "it's too easy and comfortable to do what I have always done" way of thinking. We want change to happen, but we're just not willing to do what it takes to make it happen. The problem is, this is the very thing that needs changing.

Sixty-year-old Evelyn knows just how powerful accountability can be. For several months she struggled to maintain a consistent walking routine. She knew it was something she should do, but she wasn't committed to making it happen. There was never enough time or she was not feeling up to it. It reached a point where I thought she had become too comfortable making excuses.

It wasn't until Evelyn left town several months ago that she realized her need for more accountability. She asked me if she could text me after she exercised, and I said it would be fine. Once she reached her destination, Evelyn didn't miss a workout. The irresponsibility of not living up to her end of the bargain was unacceptable to her. The thought of making more excuses for not walking had become distressing. She has continued the texting practice with me ever since.

3. We lack the confidence needed to change.

We allow failed past experiences to get in the way of our desire to change. If only change were easier, we would be the person we always wanted to be. We would have the job, relationships, and health we have always dreamed of.

However, that's not how it works. Change is hard because it requires all of you. It demands full- on commitment and dedication. It diminishes your weaknesses and empowers your motivation and resolve. You will learn more about yourself than you ever thought possible. That is the very essence of change.

The encouraging and uplifting words of a friend or family member can be all it takes to improve morale and turn things around. When you leverage your success in accomplishing small tasks into taking on larger tasks, the momentum for change gains steam. Confidence is then in place for the more challenging areas that you want to change.

With her weight around 300 pounds, Gayle epitomized how a lack of confidence will destroy efforts to improve wellness. Several times throughout the course of a workout she would say, "I can't do this" or would make excuses about why she should not try something more challenging. As a result, Gayle made very little progress. The same was true with her diet; anytime self-control was needed she chose immediate gratification.

At one point, Gayle had cancelled her scheduled workouts with me a staggering ten times in a row. Her self-defeating attitude empowered her lack of desire. This became a vicious cycle which inevitably led to the termination of her wellness program.

4. We establish the "societal norm" routine.

We settle for what society dictates rather than what is best for us. Society says a poor diet, sedentary lifestyle, and stressful day-to-day living are the normal American way of life. As a result, our health has suffered greatly. This has led us to record levels of obesity, diabetes, and heart disease and resulting strokes, metabolic syndrome, cancer, joint pain, and even discrimination.

Sixty-four-year-old Deborah is the poster child for the "societal norm." Suckered by the strength of advertisements and with her ways set in concrete, Deborah never opens herself up to change. She lets the people with the most "authority" dictate how she views most of life's topics and issues. Deborah believes everything she hears about an advertised product or medication without questioning it. This naive and closed-off approach doesn't allow for any growth whatsoever, regardless of her unique, individual needs. She brushes off any compelling evidence that contradicts her own health and wellness philosophy, because society in general "knows" what's best.

Sadly, Deborah is not alone in her thinking. I have other clients with similar beliefs but I chose Deborah because she is on several different medications and refuses to do anything about health beyond taking medication.

If it hurts, take a pill; if a blood level is out of range, take a pill; and if you're sick, take a pill—with no regard to the potential consequences. Why? Because that is what we are told to do.

CHAPTER QUESTIONS:

1. What does wellness mean to you?

Able to sleep & wake w/o pain

Able to run/walk

No need for medicines that offer tradeoffs like — you won't have A-fib, but you'll feel like you're carrying around 25 extra lbs.

2. What changes are you willing to make in order to meet that definition?

Exercise more. Give up sugar & refined grains

Exercise w/ more intensity

3. On a scale of 1-10, what is your level of confidence that you can make the changes you need to make to be well?

7

CHAPTER 4
YOU: YOUR OWN WORST ENEMY?

"I just never thought that could happen to me."
– Denise

When do you perform your best? When you're stressed-out to the max or totally at ease? Are you up on a stage in front of many, or in the quiet of your home unseen? Do you have to reach wits' end before you perform your best?

Discovering how you handle adversity relating to your wellness is imperative if you want to succeed in a long-term plan. The way in which we overcome adversity speaks directly to the strength of our individual mental and spiritual characteristics. These characteristics create the strength of our resolve. When we *know* our meaning and purpose in life and associate what is most important to us with our goals, we are best prepared for whatever life has to offer.

The following is what I call the **Eight KNOWS of Your Wellness**. Each **KNOW** speaks directly to adversity as it affects your wellness program. Any one or more of these issues can wreak havoc with your plan to get healthier. They can stand in the way of starting a program or ending one that is in full motion. Having a greater understanding of yourself and using the **Eight KNOWS of Your Wellness** to leverage your program will reduce your chance of falling prey to societal norms, unrealistic expectations, and a lack of desire—all of which can lead to the end of your self-care program.

1. **KNOW Your Body** – Susan, 66, had been complaining about hip pain for several months, but it never seemed to bother her while she was working out in the gym or playing racquetball three times a week. The only time she hurt was during walks of two miles or longer. At first, Susan was convinced that her pain required surgery, but after several doctor visits she concluded no surgery was needed. Instead, after only a few sessions with a physical therapist, Susan was as good as new.

   Many people who experience pain have no idea what is going on in their bodies. How well do you know your body? Knowing your body from a pain and energy standpoint is a good place to start. The more attuned you are to your body, the better you can assess its efficiency and identify its weaknesses. When you reach this awareness, you are able to meet your body's needs and can better answer the question "Is my injury something that time will heal or is it more serious?"

   This same body awareness applies to your energy level. I am convinced that some people neglect their self-care for so long that they can no longer recall what having energy feels like. Over time, their energy has waned to the point that this lower energy level has become their "normal."

   On a scale of 1 to 10, 10 being the highest, what is your energy level right now? How is it different from what it was ten, fifteen, and twenty years ago?

Knowing what your body is capable of doing also helps set limits on your goals. An over-zealous approach can lead to injury, burnout, and feeling overwhelmed. That deflates your motivation and reduces your chance of reaching your goals. Plan carefully!

2. **KNOW Your Will** – Imagine a scale from 1 to 10, with 1 being a very low will and 10 being very high. We all fall somewhere on that scale and our numbers are directly related to where we feel most comfortable.

    Jason, 29, works as a physician's assistant in a general practitioner's office. He wants to be well using preventative measures such as maintaining low stress levels, regular exercise, and proper work/life balance. Although he is not consistent with the fitness norms for adequate exercise frequency and duration, Jason regularly exercises. He lifts weights every Wednesday for 30 to 45 minutes and walks 2 to 3 miles at 3.0 to 3.5 mph on a treadmill every Tuesday and Thursday morning. This is the routine with which he is most comfortable. He is not willing to add another day or two or increase the level of intensity of either his weight training or walking workouts. Jason clearly has a strong will to follow through with his routine week in and week out, but he is fixed on the amount he will do and will not try doing more.

    How true is the statement "If there's a will, there's a way"? When we really want something, we are going to take whatever measures necessary to get it. Developing your will in things that are health-promoting and life-giving will go a long way towards enhancing your quality of life. Recall the last thing you wanted. Did you do everything (within reason) you could to attain it? On a scale of 1–10, what is your will in regards to keeping your regular doctor's appointments, achieving a better food intake, or getting adequate sleep at night? What would it take to bump one of these up to the next number on that scale?

3. **KNOW Your Confidence** – My oldest daughter, Brittany, was listed as a finalist for a PTA-sponsored art reception for the sixth grade. At the reception there were drawings, photographs, poetry, and music compositions on display from over two hundred sixth-, seventh-, and eighth-graders. Impressive! Brittany said, "Dad, I think I'm going to win a ribbon or a trophy." I thought, "Uh-oh!" I didn't want her to get her hopes up too high; there was some impressive talent on display. When they got to the sixth-graders and read off the names of the three Honorable Mentions, no Brittany. Then, Third Place—no Brittany. I was really getting nervous. Then, "Second Place . . . Brittany Gregory." I was so excited I was about to jump out of my skin. Afterwards, Brittany said, "I've never won anything like this before." She had never won anything before, but she expected to win. Usually, expectations of winning come from winning. Not this time. Do you expect to "win" regardless of your past?

The greater your confidence, the greater the effort you will put forth and the better you will get at what you do. So, how do you increase your confidence? First, start setting small S.M.A.R.T. goals (Chapter 5) that apply to your wellness plan and work your way up to bigger ones. It's the little victories that increase your confidence in meeting the larger goals. Second, draw upon your strengths in past experiences when you were successful, then apply those strengths to your goals. For example, display self-control at work on a regular basis and then transfer that self-control to your food intake at home.

4. **KNOW What Works Best For You** – It was Easter Sunday, and my kids, David, Lauren, and Brittany, were going through their Easter baskets. When David, age 6, had finished with his basket, he said, "I don't believe in this bunny carrying a bunch of eggs story. It's Mom and Dad who are doing all of this."

I said, "Santa Claus and the Easter Bunny only bring toys and goodies to those who believe in them." Lauren responded, "Yeah, you can't believe in Santa Claus and not the Easter Bunny."

David quickly and emphatically replied, "Oh, come on—that's totally different." Because Santa Claus had more to offer, he made sense for David. Anything less would not suffice.

What do you know about what works best for you? How might brainstorming help you? Knowing your strengths, limitations, resources, and support systems will assist you in choosing the right time and type of exercise to perform, the right place to shop for healthy foods, the right balance between your work and family/social life, and so much more. Not knowing what works best for you causes wellness program chaos.

My job as a personal trainer is to find what works best for my clients in their exercise programs. Discovering what works best in the other areas of their wellness is left up to them. As a wellness coach, I guide them through a process towards breakthrough by asking the right questions and assisting them in constructing their goals.

5. **KNOW Your Strengths** – Did you notice that there isn't a KNOW for weaknesses? There is absolutely no reason to exploit your shortcomings; instead, let's exalt your strengths. Identify your strengths, then apply them to your health, fitness, and wellness

plan. Are you disciplined? Do you have self-control? Is patience one of your strengths? Recall an experience in your past where you used your strengths and were successful. How did that feel?

Cynthia, 46, one of my former coaching clients, discovered just how to apply her professional strengths to balance her work and family life. For years, she missed her kids' homework time, volleyball games, and piano recitals. A very strong personality, Cynthia transferred her ability to communicate with her work team, and her time management skills, to her family life. She did this by delegating the oversight of two large projects to a colleague, which greatly reduced her extra work time. This allowed her to spend more time with her family and lessen the stress that all of the family members were experiencing due to her frequent absence. She became more empathetic towards her husband and children, which led to stronger relationships and ultimately a more relaxed home environment.

6. **KNOW Your Opportunities** – and take advantage of them. If a group wants you to join them for a pick-up basketball game, go for it. If you have been trying to get your husband to exercise more and he suggests going for a walk, jump on it. Whatever it is, don't miss out. Be open to new ideas and possibilities.

People who practice self-care regularly tend to look for ways to get healthier. For those who are not presently caring for their health, acting on wellness opportunities becomes more of a challenge. I have met many people throughout the years in my personal training business who believe they should lose weight before they start exercising. Be it embarrassment in the gym because of their low fitness levels or excessive weight, people often think the gym is a place where only healthy and fit people go. The opposite is true—the gym is an opportunity.

Kenneth was sedentary, fifty pounds overweight, and had elevated blood pressure, cholesterol, and triglyceride levels. He accepted his doctor's recommendation to begin a workout program. At first, Kenneth was reluctant to try anything. He performed only our scheduled workouts. Once he realized some of the benefits of his twice-a-week resistance-training regimen, though, he began asking about other fitness opportunities available around town. After scanning the Internet and local newspaper, Kenneth decided to join a running group that used a marathon training program. Five months later, Kenneth ran his first marathon at the age of fifty-four. In the past seven years, Kenneth has run many marathons, ridden on bike rides of 100 miles or longer, and now regularly attends yoga and Pilates classes. And, Kenneth has maintained his resistance training workouts. To this day, his doctor continues to give him a thumbs-up report due to his weight loss and lower blood pressure, cholesterol, and triglyceride counts. His increased fitness activities also affected his food intake. His diet has become much healthier, and he is always looking for something new and healthy to try.

7. **KNOW What's Realistic For You** – Nine years ago, my wife told my daughter Lauren, then five years old, that she couldn't do something she wanted to do. Lauren ran inside, grabbed her overnight bag, threw underwear and a toothbrush in it, and ran out the door. She darted across the yard and down the street to her friend Julie's house saying, "I'm running away." I got home about an hour later and walked down to Julie's house to get her for supper. When we got home, everyone was at the dinner table. She told me, "Dad, I'm going to run away."

I responded, "Okay, but you know you will have to drop out of school (kindergarten) and get a job."

Lauren replied, "No, I don't. Julie's parents will pay for everything."

I said, "No, Honey, that's not the way it works!" Lauren had no realistic view about how the world operates.

Do you have realistic expectations of who you can be regarding your wellness? Recalling your past experiences of success will help you set realistic, attainable goals. Unrealistic goals usually lead to frustration, disappointment, and, ultimately, the end of a self-care program. People often expect greater returns on their investment than is realistic, instead of being patient and enjoying what benefits they do receive for their hard work.

What steps can you put in place to avoid falling into this trap?

8. **KNOW Your Dreams** – Keeping your dreams in the forefront of your mind helps you stay focused on the long-term vision you have set. Dreams define you and establish your destination: who and where you want to be. Knowing your will answers the question "What do I want right now?" Knowing your dreams answers the ultimate question of who you want to become.

   Denise, 31, had never mentioned her wellness dreams to me. We had been training for several months when she realized where all her hard work could ultimately lead. She had seen her blood profile improve and felt an increase in energy and confidence. Then Denise went clothes shopping one afternoon. At her next session, our conversation went something like this: "I haven't lost that much weight, but never in my wildest dreams did I think that I could fit into a size 12." I replied, "As you have been dropping body fat, you have been adding muscle, hence the slower weight loss."

   She said, "I know, I just never thought that could happen to me."

Dreams require a positive and exhilarating outlook regarding the future. They have a way of moving people to action because of the possibilities and energy that they create. Dreams encourage your full engagement. An all-inspired effort will empower your will and resolve as you perform the task at hand. Self-care coupled with a dream is tough to beat.

ROADBLOCKS AND REASONS

Human behavior really intrigues me. Why do we do what we do? So often we are destructive to both ourselves and those around us. This phenomenon seems to be strongest in the area of self-care. Learning coping mechanisms and ways to combat apathy are powerful strategies for overcoming the unfortunate circumstances that tend to arise at moment's notice. When you have an alternate plan in place, your chances for successfully completing your wellness goals increase significantly.

Here is a list of roadblocks and reasons that I hear on a regular basis when I ask people why they don't take better care of themselves. The list addresses short-term and long-term life issues, as well as self-destructive reasoning. Which, if any, do you identify with?

ROADBLOCKS (Life Issues)

1. **Relationships** – When family members need our help, sometimes giving that help interferes with a wellness activity we planned, such as a stress-relieving massage. This is a great time to brainstorm. Generate other ways to relieve your stress so you can accomplish all you need to do. In place of the massage appointment, try a hot bath, a massage by your spouse, drinking a glass of wine while listening to relaxing music, or watching a beautiful sunset— examples of other strong relaxation techniques.

   When you brainstorm wellness activities, always remember to include all of the ideas that come to mind, regardless of how outlandish they might sound. You never know what useful ideas may come from what first seems to be a ridiculous thought.

2. **Illness/Injury** – Illnesses and injuries happen, even to the healthiest of us. It's not uncommon for me to get a phone call or text from a client who has injured herself at home or at her job. When you're injured or ill, it's a good time to skip a few workouts and get healthy again. Allowing your body the rest it needs to recover is always better than forcing your way through a workout or eating even healthy foods when your stomach may not be ready for them.

3. **Failed, or No, Support Systems** – When friends and family members don't support each other's efforts to exercise, eat right, and practice general self-care, it becomes exponentially more difficult to follow through on any wellness program. A little bit of support and encouragement go a long way in helping someone take care of himself or herself. If you are not currently in a support group, join one that is supportive of your new healthy behavior (such as a running group, fitness boot camp, or neighborhood walking friends). These groups increase your responsibility and accountability to the commitments you make for a healthier life.

4. **Time Limitations** – It happens to us all: an unexpected meeting at work; a car breaks down; one child has choir practice, another basketball practice, and your third child is at home sick. All are legitimate reasons for running out of time.

5. **Financial Struggles** – Any time money is short, things get cut from the spending side of the ledger. Unfortunately, healthy practices are among the first to go. Healthy foods (which are typically more expensive), workout facilities, massage appointments, yoga classes, and wellness coaching sessions

hit the chopping block. Yet, it is during these stressful financial times when you most need health-promoting activities.

6. **Limited Resources** – There is always a way to create a healthy environment around you, even when your resources may be restricted. The availability of money, equipment, and facilities can affect your program. Plan accordingly! Instead of planning how to work within their newly limited resources, some clients have "accidentally" left their clothes at home so they cannot work out. What could they have done instead?

7. **Lack of Motivation** – I have had people tell me that they just didn't want to work out at the time of their appointment, so they didn't. Most of the time, people will cite another reason to give their excuse legitimacy, but I often sense it's really a lack of desire.

8. **Resistance** – Some people hit lock-down mode within conventional wisdom and resist being open to different ideas. This is never more evident to me than in discussing dietary information. It's so easy to get set in your ways when all you ever believe is one angle of a topic, especially when it sounds "right." A willingness to learn and try new things leads to fresh possibilities and opportunities.

9. **Skepticism** – Are the benefits worth the effort and sacrifice? Weighing the pros and cons of any issue requires getting enough information to make an informed decision. Where can you go to learn more about the decision you are making?

SELF-DESTRUCTIVE REASONING

1. *It's all good.* — Illness happens only to others. I'm disease-free; I must be healthy and well.

2. *There's nothing fun about sacrifice and deprivation.* — I am going to eat and do whatever I want.

3. *I'm too stressed.* — A preoccupation with the stressor often leads to poor dietary choices and inactivity. That preoccupation presents a challenge to stress management. Frequently, under stress, we abandon any and all healthy living.

4. *I'm depressed.* — If severe enough, this mental state leads to apathy and lethargy.

5. *What are all of these wellness activities going to do for me?* — Being convinced that something is good for you starts with information. Educate yourself!

6. *Health is not on my priority list . . . until I don't have it anymore.* — The saying "An ounce of prevention is worth a pound of cure" is never more relevant than here. Gaining an understanding of what health issues other people your age, sex, and race are experiencing is important.

7. *I was never an athlete nor did I have to practice healthy behaviors before.* — A healthy lifestyle has nothing to do with your non-athletic background or unhealthy living in the past. It's NEVER too late to start.

8. *I'll do it later!* — Many times, people will continue to procrastinate about taking care of themselves until a health crisis arrives.

9. *I don't want to.* — People have to want to practice self-care in order to do so.

10. *I can't do it! Changing my routine is too hard!* — Most people won't try if they lack the confidence to succeed. This is often the result of failed attempts in the past.

11. *I'm not ready, willing, or able!* — Spouses, quit nagging! The more you nag, the farther away you drive the other person. Resistance is at work here; nobody wants to be told what to do. Eliminate judgmental statements and guilt trips. Don't make demands or give ultimatums.

12. *Give me all of the health advice and I'll make my own decisions. There are some things I refuse to give up.* — Some people will reject any information that is given to them. Or they pick and choose the information that best suits their willingness to change.

I hope that by now you are realizing that a wellness program starts between the ears. So much of what we do is based on our readiness, willingness, and belief that we *can* do it. By getting to know ourselves better, we can anticipate and prepare for times when adversity strikes our well-being or disrupts or plans. Having an alternate plan ready to work through our own roadblocks and self-destructive reasoning will strengthen our resolve when the unfortunate happens. Alternate plans keep us on the straight and narrow road to reaching our best selves.

CHAPTER QUESTIONS:

1. Which KNOWS of Your Wellness would you like to explore at greater length?

2. What roadblocks are you facing regarding your self-care?

3. What will you do to overcome those roadblocks?

CHAPTER 5
CREATING A VISION & S.M.A.R.T. GOALS

Setting goals activates motivation around things that are most important to you.

In Chapters 5 and 6, I draw on what I learned from Wellcoaches, a certified health and wellness coaching program based in Wellesley, Massachusetts (www.Wellcoaches.com), as well as from my own experiences with my clients.

Do you recall, from the preface, my client Michael and his incredible weight loss? Many things led to Michael's success, but none was more important than his vision. At the beginning of his program, Michael outlined to me what he saw himself doing. He followed that up with giving me a day-to-day, week-to-week, and month-to-month forecast of his immediate and long-term vision. That forecast proved to be the biggest predictor of his success.

VISIONS

Visions describe a desirable future that inspires and motivates us. A vision answers the question "What is my best self?" Or, "What is my best possible situation?" Visions are energizing and life-giving. They give you direction and propel your growth. Visions also help generate a sense of urgency because of their ability to motivate. In my coaching practice, the first thing I have my clients do is design a wellness vision. Helping them stay focused on that vision is the very nature of my coaching.

Without visions, life becomes stale and boring. One of the major reasons we fail to meet our goals stems from not having a clear vision. First, we must have a destination in mind, and then plan how to get there. In the words of the philosopher Epictetus, "First say to yourself what you would be; then do what you have to do."[1] That's exactly how a vision works. Decide where you want to be months or years down the road, then work backwards by setting goals to help you get there.

Mary, 52, always saw her New Year's resolutions fade away by mid-February. She halfheartedly addressed her plan of action, thinking it would take care of itself. Usually, Mary's resolutions were the same: exercise more, make necessary dietary changes, and become better organized. No thought of a vision and no written, specific goals do not make a sound approach to changing your life. Then, about two and a half years ago, Mary did make a change. During our first coaching session, she developed her wellness vision and set three-month and weekly S.M.A.R.T. goals that laid the foundation for her future success. She is now flourishing: setting and meeting challenging goals on a weekly basis.

Take a look at your dream, your personal wellness vision. Remember, this is YOUR desire for a healthier you, not someone else's for you. Ultimately, a wellness vision is a statement of who you want to be. It answers the question "What healthy, energizing, and life-giving behaviors do I want to practice consistently?" Use the following questions[2] to develop your vision.

1. *A Look into the Future* — What kind of person do you want to be regarding your health, fitness, and/or wellness? If you were to become your best, well self, what would you look and feel like? What behaviors would you be performing regularly?

2. *Important Factors* — What are the most important factors of your wellness vision? How will you stay on course when you encounter challenges? On a scale of 1–10, how significant are each of those factors to you?

3. *Past Experiences* — What have been your best experiences with the most significant factors of your vision?

4. *Values* — Which of your values are supported by your vision?

5. *Motivators* — What are all of the benefits of you reaching your wellness vision?

6. *Desire* — How hard are you willing to work to reach your vision?

7. *Distance* — Right now, how far are you from reaching your vision?

8. *Confidence* — On a scale of 1–10, how confident are you that you will reach your vision? How realistic is your vision?

9. *Challenges* — What could get in the way of you reaching your vision?

10. *Strengths* — How can you apply what you have learned from past successes to meet potential challenges ahead?

11. *Support Systems* — Who can support you as you journey towards your vision? How can your environments and situations assist or hurt you along the way?

12. *Alternate Plans* — What strategies can you put in place to counter potential challenges?

S.M.A.R.T. GOAL-SETTING

Now, it's time to start setting goals. We set goals in order to measure our progress; the **S.M.A.R.T.**er we design our goals, the greater our chance of success. The beauty of the goal-setting technique I am about to describe is that it applies to all areas of life, not just to your health, fitness, and wellness. George T. Doran created S.M.A.R.T. goals[3] in 1981 to aid business managers, but Doran's S.M.A.R.T. goals are now used in many other settings. I have seen people set professional, organizational, even child-rearing goals using this format, and it works!

Here's the successful goal-setting equation:

S.M.A.R.T. Goal + Your Values (attached to the goal) + Accountability + Desire to Change = ULTIMATE SUCCESS

First, let's take a look at what the acronym S.M.A.R.T. stands for.

Specific
Making a goal as specific as possible is imperative to its success.

Measurable
When a goal is measurable, it allows for monitoring its success.

Action-Driven/Achievable/Attainable
In your mind's eye, you should be able to see yourself performing your goal.

Realistic/Relevant
Your goal should be realistic and challenging and pertinent to your vision.

Timely/Tangible
Your goal should always have a start and end date/time.

To begin the goal-setting process, brainstorm different ideas about healthy behaviors you would like to perform on a regular basis to help you reach your best self. Go back to Chapter 1 and answer the question "What makes you feel most alive?" Don't you want more of that? What is it going to take to get there? Then, consider what actions you will do in the first week to get the ball rolling in that direction. This is a time to generate ideas and lay the foundation for your future goals.

Envisioning our wellness becomes less overwhelming when we break it down into manageable steps. These steps are the building blocks to reaching the vision that we seek to attain. After all, no marathon has ever been run without taking the first step. So, by making small changes every day towards our wellness vision we will experience the benefits of living a life of wellness has to offer. Setting S.M.A.R.T. goals allows us to activate our motivations toward those things that are most important to us.

Once you have a good idea about what you want to do, begin the S.M.A.R.T. goal-writing process with the phrase "I will . . . . " The first goals you write should be three-month goals. These are goals that refer to behaviors you want to be practicing consistently three months from now. Weekly goals include the daily steps to get there. For example, if you are currently sedentary and would like to increase your bone density to reduce your risk of osteoporosis, you might state your three-month goal as, "I will perform three forty-five-minute strength-training sessions per week on Monday, Wednesday, and Friday at 8 a.m." The first week of this three-month period might include the goal "I will perform one thirty-minute strength-training session this week on Wednesday at 8 a.m." No more than four three-month S.M.A.R.T. goals should be set at the beginning of each three-month period.

Establishing three-month and weekly S.M.A.R.T. *behavioral* goals are *essential* to help you take the small steps necessary to reach your vision. Well designed goals are always behavioral, which means, these goals are what you *do*, not what *happens* when you do the behaviors.

For example, a goal of "I will walk for thirty minutes, Monday through Friday, at 8 a.m." will help you reach the outcome (your vision) of increasing your energy. Outcomes of completed goals should be stated in your vision, not stated as goals.

Once you have set your S.M.A.R.T. goals, find an accountability partner to help you see them through. When we allow another person to hold us accountable for our goals, we increase the likelihood of accomplishing those goals. Having someone to answer to forces us to be responsible and accountable for our actions and inactions. It can be quite uncomfortable to tell your partner that you didn't do what you said you would.

GIMME AN "S"

Let's start breaking down the S.M.A.R.T. way to write goals.

As I thumb through my thesaurus (not really—it's on my computer, but isn't that cool?), I see that *specificity*, which represents the **S** in S.M.A.R.T., is a synonym for *exact* and *explicit*. The importance of designing goals is to make them as exact and explicit as possible. This will help reduce the ambiguity that often surrounds our goals. Specific goals describe in detail what is going to happen.

Here are a few examples of poorly written goals. Following each one is the S.M.A.R.T. goal direction that it fails to follow:

1. I am going to lose weight. **SPECIFICITY**

2. I want to get healthier. **MEASURABLE**

3. I need to smoke less. **ACTION-DRIVEN**

4. I am going to run a marathon next month. **REALISTIC/RELEVANT**

5. I want to relax more. **TIMELY/TANGIBLE**

Let's take a look at the first one, "I am going to lose weight." To begin with, remember that all goals should start with the words "I will . . . ."

This commits you, while the "I want to," "I need to," and "I am going to" don't provide that commitment. Also, weight loss should never be a goal; it is an outcome. It is a result of meeting other goals that lead to weight loss, such as those associated with your diet.

The specificity of a goal means that goal answers the questions "Who? What? When? Where? Why?" and "How?" When all of these questions are answered in the goal, the goal has specificity. Specific goals give us direction and help us to stay focused on what we have set out to accomplish.

If spending more quality time with your family is in your wellness vision (outcome), an example of goal-setting to reach that vision would be:

> **GOAL:** I will leave work at 5 p.m. Monday through Friday this week.
>
> **COMMENT:** I will get to work an hour earlier every day this week so that I can leave work to spend more time with my family.
>
> **GOAL:** I will speak with my wife this Wednesday evening at 7 p.m. to plan several family excursions and trips for the next three months.
>
> **COMMENT:** This will create a greater balance between my work and family life.

Both of these goals are specific. You can actually see yourself executing these goals. As a result, movement and action soon take place. When goals provide a clear picture of what we want, it is easy to get ourselves moving. The comment after each goal gives additional information without making the goal too long and drawn-out.

GIMME AN "M"

Setting goals activates motivation toward the things that are most important to you. Concrete actions within your goal facilitate reaching that goal. The **M** of the S.M.A.R.T. acronym represents making your goals *measurable*. All too often our goals are vague, and we can't measure our progress. A goal that is measurable is one that answers the questions "How much? How many? How often? How intense? How long?" and "How will I know when I have completed the goal?" Not all of these questions need an answer, but you should be able to answer at least one question per goal. If you leave the question(s) unanswered, you will have no clear route to success.

According to Bob Tschannen-Moran of LifeTrekCoaching.com, measures "could be used both before and after we achieve the goal. They support both the action and the maintenance stages of change. It's great to identify measures that can become a permanent part of your routine. That's why people use pillboxes, for example: at a glance, it's easy to answer the question 'Did I take my pills today?' We don't use that measure just while we are learning to take our pills. We use that measure forever, because it assists us to stay on track." [4]

For example, the poorly written goal "I want to get healthier" is not a measurable goal. How is it possible to measure when you are "healthier"? It is also important to design goals stating what you will do, not what you won't do. Remember to always start your goal with "I will . . . ," to show strong commitment to a specific action. Here are a couple of good goal examples:

> **GOAL:** I will eat one cup of Rocky Road ice cream on Friday after dinner this week.
> COMMENT: One cup is down from the usual five cups a week that I normally eat.
>
> **GOAL:** I will write three things that I am grateful for in my gratitude journal at 8 p.m. every night this week.

COMMENT: This will help me stay focused on the things that are most important to me and help reduce stress in my life.

Both of these goals are easy to evaluate. To determine your level of success, calculate what percentage of the goal you have completed. If you achieve less than 60% of your goal, the goal may be too difficult. When you reach 100% of your goal, commit to setting a more challenging goal. Remember, it's important to keep your goals short and to the point, so you will know when you have reached your destination.

GIMME AN "A"

As we make our way through the S.M.A.R.T. acronym, I hope your understanding of goals becomes clearer and more concise; that will aid your focus and direction.

Depending upon whom you talk to, the **A** in S.M.A.R.T. stands for *action-driven, achievable*, and/or *attainable*. I prefer *action-driven* because the other two apply more to how realistic the goal is. Clearly, if your goal is written in a way that encompasses these things, your chances of accomplishing that goal increase. Like specificity, a goal that is action-driven is one that you can see being performed. This enhances your chance of completing the task at hand. Painting a clear picture of what it is you will be doing is imperative for success.

The example goal "I need to smoke less" is not an action-based goal. How can you see yourself *not doing* something? Instead, naming a substitute activity, such as chewing gum or taking a walk in lieu of smoking, would be a good, action-based anti-smoking goal.

The fact that you currently smoke will determine whether or not your "need" to stop smoking is achievable. I point out the word "need" because smoking cessation is not a need; it's a strategy to meet your need of physical well-being. The goal "I need to smoke less" is not an action-based goal. The phrase "smoke less" is not specific enough; it does not give the details of the goal being set. *What* is it that you will be doing? Providing these details creates greater focus, commitment, and motivation to meet your goal.

You also reduce the probability that you will "accidentally" set a goal that is too high when you follow the necessary steps in developing your wellness vision, three-month S.M.A.R.T. goals, and weekly S.M.A.R.T. goals. Answer the following questions when you write your goals to help you set action-based, achievable goals.

1. Can I see myself performing this goal?

2. On a scale of 1 to 10, 10 being the highest, what is my confidence level that I will complete this goal?

3. On a scale of 1 to 10, 10 being the highest, what priority does this goal have in my life?

4. Am I willing to do what it takes to complete this goal?

5. Is everything in place for me to meet this goal (such as time, finances, support from others, work, and family life)?

Here are some examples of action-based goals. Ask yourself the five previous questions for each goal to see how the goals measure up.

> **GOAL:** I will chew a piece of gum every time I feel the urge to smoke on Monday, Wednesday, and Friday this week.
>
> **COMMENT:** I currently try to willpower my way through self-denial, which has not been very successful.

> **GOAL:** I will take a brisk walk around my neighborhood every time I feel the urge to smoke on Tuesday, Thursday, and Saturday this week.
>
> **COMMENT:** I currently try to willpower my way through self-denial, which has not been very successful.

GIMME AN "R"

How are you doing so far? Are your goals specific, measurable, and action-based? How about realistic and relevant? As with the **A** in the S.M.A.R.T. acronym, the **R** has two references, depending on which discussion of S.M.A.R.T. goals you read: *realistic* or *relevant*. Both elements are essential to successful goal-setting.

Realistic – How successful do you think you are going to be if your goals are unrealistic? The word *unrealistic* elicits non-real images, and inabilities. I see it all the time with my new personal training clients; their initial expectations are far beyond the speed of change that the body can experience. This reality often brings them back down to earth and a realistic approach often ensues. Goals that are poorly written in this way are often thought to be non-specific, but in fact the goal is *both* unrealistic *and* non-specific. For example, "I am going to run a marathon next month" is unrealistic if you are currently sedentary. Breaking that goal into many smaller, realistic goals is the recipe for success. Ask yourself the following questions:

1. Do I honestly believe that I can complete this goal?

2. Are my finances, the environment around me, and the time available conducive for my meeting this goal?

3. Is a strong social support system needed to be successful with this goal? How is my social support, right now?

4. Am I willing to make the sacrifices needed to complete this goal?

Relevant – There's nothing like relevance when it comes to goals. Each day, week, month, even year builds on the previous one when goals are relevant. In goal-setting, starting with "baby steps," followed by "adolescent steps," and then "adult steps" will lead to increased confidence and success in reaching your goals and visions. In their first few visits, my personal training clients ALWAYS start with less work than they are capable of handling and progress very slowly. This not only prevents injury, but it also makes each workout relevant for the next workout and builds confidence along the way. Ask yourself the following questions:

1. Is my goal the next step towards my three-month goal or wellness vision?

2. How pertinent is my goal to what I really want?

3. Is completing my goal going to give me the confidence I need to set a more challenging goal next week?

4. What will I learn from successfully completing this goal?

The poorly written goal example "I am going to run a marathon next month" may not be realistic or relevant. If you are currently sedentary, running a marathon is not only unrealistic, it is downright ridiculous. However, if you are an avid runner, running a marathon may be a reasonable goal for next month. And, if your main objective is to be generally fit, running a marathon is a bit of overkill. You can reach a high level of fitness without having to run a marathon that may take a toll on your body. Running shorter distances may be more relevant to what you are trying to accomplish.

If general fitness goal-setting is of interest to you, consider the four questions above when you construct your plan. Here are several example goals that are realistic and relevant.

> **GOAL:** I will attend Pilates class on Monday at 11 a.m. and Thursday at 3 p.m. this week.
> COMMENT: This is *realistic* for me because I currently attend one class a week.

> **GOAL:** I will run 3 miles on Monday, Wednesday, Friday, and Saturday at 6 a.m.

COMMENT: This is *relevant* to my three-month goal of running a half-marathon.

GIMME A "T"

We always need to remember why we are setting goals in the first place: to stay focused and on track and to lead us to our vision. It is easy to get lost in the goal-setting process and forget our primary motivation if our goals are not specific, measurable, action-driven, realistic/relevant, and timely/tangible. As you set your goals, always remember what is most important to you right now.

The **T** refers to two qualities, too: *timely* and *tangible*. You can follow all of the rules we have talked about regarding S.M.A.R.T. goals, but if you leave out the time and tangibility factor, you can kiss those goals goodbye! Including a completion date with your goal gives you a sense of urgency and encourages immediate action. Setting a reasonable time frame also helps make sense of your goal. If you set an unrealistic timetable, you probably won't take the goal seriously.

The poorly written goal example "I want to relax more" is neither timely nor tangible. For a goal to be tangible, it needs to have a physical presence, something that can be detected by at least one of the senses. When a goal is tangible, it becomes easier to measure and achieve. When you design your goal, ask yourself the following timely/tangible questions:

1. When am I going to complete this goal?

2. How much time will be involved in reaching this goal?

3. Can I "see" myself, with one of the five senses, performing this goal?

4. Can I observe this goal with my senses or is it imaginary?

If relaxation is a goal, consider the four questions above when you construct your plan. Here are some example goals that are *timely* and *tangible*. They provide a time in which the activity is to take place and an activity that can be experienced by one of the senses.

> **GOAL:** I will schedule a one-hour massage for 5 p.m. on Friday.
>
> COMMENT: This will help me relax after a long week at the office.

> **GOAL:** I will take a hot bath every night (M–F) this week at 8 p.m.
>
> COMMENT: It will help reduce stress to relax on a daily basis.

Consider the following when designing your vision and S.M.A.R.T. goals:

1. *What's your wellness, health, and fitness history?* Our past successes in all areas of life can be drawn upon to help us be successful with future challenges in our wellness programs.

2. *Where are you currently with your wellness, health, and fitness programs?* Thankfully, performing healthy behaviors right now does not require that you have done so in the past. By attaching what you truly value in life to S.M.A.R.T. three-month and weekly goals, you are more likely to stick with your plan.

3. *Where do you want to be regarding your wellness, health, and fitness?* Having a vision is important, really important. It will give you direction and purpose as you seek your best self.

ASSESSING YOUR GOAL COMPLETION

As I explained, in order to experience consistent success with your goals, they need to be specific, measurable, action-driven, realistic/relevant, and timely/tangible (S.M.A.R.T.). When these criteria are joined with desire and accountability, the sky is the limit. A regular weekly check-in with a coach or accountability partner to assess your goal completion can also have a profound effect on your progress.

Once you have set your goals, be sure to give each goal a level of priority and confidence. On a scale of 1–4, one being the highest priority and four being the lowest priority, what is the level of importance you will give to your goal? Also, on a scale of 1–10, with ten the highest and one the lowest, what is your level of confidence that you will meet the goal that you set? If that number is a six or lower, what changes can you make to your goal to increase that confidence to a seven or higher?

At the end of each week and the end of the three-month period, take time to determine the amount of success you had with your goals. By answering the following questions, you will be able to identify what you have learned throughout the goal-setting process, and to re-evaluate your vision. After you have answered these questions about each of your goals, apply a percentage of completion to each one.

When you succeeded in your *weekly* goal, ask:

- What factors were in place that helped me be successful with this goal?

- How does my success make me feel?

- What did I learn from this goal?

- How might I change my goal to challenge myself more?

- How can I apply the success of this goal to future goals?

When you did not complete your *weekly* goal, ask:

- What was challenging about my goal?

- Is this goal still important to me?

- How does my lack of success make me feel?

- What did I learn from this experience?

- How can I grow and get better at the goal I am trying to master?

- What changes could I make in my surroundings that would aid in my success?

- How might I change my goal to make it more attainable?

At the end of three months, re-examine your *wellness vision* and *three-month* goals:

- Is my wellness vision still important to me today?

- Are my goals getting me towards my wellness vision?

- Are there any of my three-month goals I would like to modify?

- If so, which one(s)?

- What would I like that goal to be?

Evaluating your goals is important. By assessing your progress on a regular basis you will stay focused and connected to your vision. Your learning and growth experiences will be amplified throughout the process of goal-setting as you uncover more about yourself. Evaluating goals will also help you discover how you feel when things go well and when things don't go as well as you would have liked.

ACCOUNTABILITY

You can't plan for success in a wellness program without understanding the importance of accountability. Anytime you answer to someone else about your self-care, it creates a greater sense of meaning and purpose in what you are doing. This in turn increases adherence to your program. Goals without accountability disappear over time, and motivation fades.

Accountability is powerful, so powerful that for it to work its magic it has to be wanted. If someone is holding you accountable but you don't want to be, guilt feelings or a temptation to not tell the truth often arise. However, if you welcome accountability, it has the potential to push you to a level of wellness you never imagined.

One of my duties is to hold my clients responsible for their wellness behavior because no one else will. They may be held to a certain accountability by their spouses at home, but unless they have a trainer, coach, or accountability buddy, they have no one to answer to in regards to their wellness. By applying that same level of attention, energy, and accountability to your wellness program as you do to your marriage, you greatly increase your chances of success.

Have you heard these sayings? "A true friend unbosoms freely, advises justly, assists readily, adventures boldly, takes all patiently, defends courageously, and continues a friend unchangeably" (William Penn). [5] "But friendship is precious, not only in the shade but in the sunshine of life, and thanks to a benevolent arrangement of things, the greater part of life is sunshine" (Thomas Jefferson). [6] Have you ever thought about how true these statements really are? We rely heavily on others for many reasons; one is accountability. Accountability generates a sense of responsibility, and responsibility is a force for motivation.

CHAPTER QUESTIONS:

1. What is my vision?

2. Write a well-crafted weekly S.M.A.R.T. goal.

3. Write one three-month S.M.A.R.T. goal with your vision and weekly goal in mind.

CHAPTER 6
UNDERSTANDING LIFELONG CHANGE

In order to change, we must be
"sick and tired of being sick and tired."

Frequently when I am at a party, the conversation turns to exercise, diet, and weight loss. I most often hear, "I ought to start exercising," "I need to lose weight," "I should go on a diet." These statements tend to be empty and go nowhere. The conversation would be better served if people spoke honestly about where they were in the change process, such as, "I have weighed the pros and cons of beginning an exercise program, and I'm ready to go," and "I have set my S.M.A.R.T. goals for my weight loss program and I'll be starting first thing Monday morning." These statements reveal meaningful depth, insight, and commitment.

When you get right down to it, this is what it is all about: CHANGE. Changing for the better! Throughout the change process, in any area of life, we constantly move from one aspect of doing to another. Whether it's a motivational issue or one of life's circumstances, we are moving in and out of different phases of action at any given time.

I refer to willpower, self-control, and discipline as progressive forms of transformation. With each comes a stronger commitment and desire. *Willpower* is painfully pushing that bowl of ice cream out of your reach. But, willpower is not sustainable; it is therefore ineffective for the long term. Research has shown that willpower is like a tank of gas: when you empty it in one area of your life, you don't have any left for other areas of your life—the tank is dry. *Self-control* means willfully changing your actions because you want greater good for yourself. It is a stronger commitment to change than willpower because self-control's will to do better is greater. *Discipline* is what forms the obedience to a lifestyle. IT IS WHAT YOU DO without pain, sacrifice, or regret!

Remember Michael, whose incredible eleven-month, 200-pound weight loss experience I wrote about in the Preface? Throughout Michael's journey, he often spoke of the "pebble on the road" that he feared the most: that one small slip-up that would throw him out of his rhythm. Our talks about the unexpected events (the cons) that he would encounter created a greater perspective for Michael about his concerns and allowed him to see all of the possibilities that existed for him. This continuous dialogue helped him to further analyze his barriers, or "pebbles," and therefore overcome them. For example, Michael wanted the "attaboy" and "pat on the back" that he believed he deserved. He would talk about attending a party where no one acknowledged his 50-, then 100-, then 150-, and then 200-pound weight loss. Initially disappointed and frustrated, now Michael uses those times and our conversations to intensify his motivation and drive for greater success.

How do you view change? Are you ready to make a change for the better? A closer look at who you are, what you want, what is standing in your way, and how to get around those obstacles is critical as we now explore the different phases of change.

The following depiction of change is informed by the Stages of Change Model[1] developed by James Prochaska and his colleagues at the University of Rhode Island in the late 1970s. It describes where we are at different times with our behaviors. These phases are not lip service we give to those around us to get them off our case, but our own thinking during the change process. Included in each stage's description are some strategies to help get you moving to the next step as you progress to the pinnacle of the change cycle, the "I am still doing" phase.

I CAN'T DO, OR I WON'T DO

The "I can't do" phase occurs in people who would like to change but lack the confidence to do so successfully. This is often the result of unsuccessful attempts in the past and the perception that the change is too difficult to make. Closely examining what caused roadblocks in the past, along with successful completion of smaller goals in the present, can lead to an increase in confidence.

Tina, 63, is one of my fitter clients. She has a relatively "clean" diet, run/walks 15 to 20 miles a week, lifts weights twice a week, and is always looking for ways to improve herself. But with all of her fitness success, Tina still lacks confidence from time to time. It is not uncommon for her to tell me two or three times during a workout how she can't do something, such as, finish her last set on the bench press or complete a long plank. I have also noticed that she can be hesitant to start something new, out of fear of not succeeding. Tweaking her diet here and there presents a real challenge in overcoming the "I can't do" attitude, too, but Tina keeps working at it until she gets it right.

CHAPTER QUESTIONS for "I Can't Do":

A. Which of my routines prevent me from being successful?

B. What makes it hard for me to do this new behavior?

C. What is it going to take to increase my confidence in that area?

D. What are some of the barriers associated with this behavior?

The "I won't do" phase occurs when people are not willing to change because they don't believe there is a problem with their current behavior. Becoming better informed and listing all of the pros and cons of the new behavior can help propel these people into the next phase of change. It is important to be honest when making this list. Research indicates that in order to make a sustained change in behavior, you must see the pros outweighing the cons. This phase also includes people who are unwilling to invest their time, money, and/or effort in changing, even in the midst of illness or injury.

Kyle, 56, is the husband of one of my longtime training and coaching clients. My client has been trying to get Kyle to exercise for years, but to no avail. It's a pretty typical story: he was a runner when they met and courted, but stopped running shortly after they got married. He completed a marathon and decided that he had done everything in the area of running he wanted to do, so he quit. Through the years, none of Kyle's numerous aches, pains, and illnesses (bad knee, back, colds, the flu) due to not taking care of himself could propel him into starting a wellness program. The "I won't do" attitude had a crippling affect on his ability to move forward with any kind of self-care plan.

CHAPTER QUESTIONS for "I Won't Do":

A. What are the benefits of changing my behavior?

B. Where can I get more information on the benefits of living a healthy lifestyle?

C. How is my current behavior affecting my health?

D. If I continue with this unhealthy behavior, how will it affect my health years from now?

I MIGHT DO

The "I might do" phase occurs when a person considers starting a new behavior within the next six months. These people are often more aware of problems that they have than those in the "I can't do" and "I won't do" phase. The cons are more important than the pros during this time because the person has low confidence in his or her ability to start and maintain a new healthy behavior. Also, people in "I might do" have not yet discovered that one legitimate reason why they should be engaging in a new behavior.

People do best when they connect what they value with their wellness and fitness goals. When you add that to additional information regarding the benefits of the new, desired behavior, you get a highly motivated and confident person willing to give it her all. However, to get to that point, you must find the one or more valid reason(s) needed to set the ball in motion.

Olivia, 42, is currently in the "I might do" phase with her food intake. Needing to lose about fifty pounds, Olivia is still not sure that the bang is worth the buck. For her, many of life's pleasures come from eating food containing large amounts of sugar. Presently, she is free of pain and disease, but Olivia understands that in order to lose the weight the doctors tell her to lose, she must change her diet. This is where her ambivalence begins. We are constantly talking about the benefits of eating better and the consequences of staying the same. As of today, Olivia's cons are winning, but the pros are gaining ground.

CHAPTER QUESTIONS for "I Might Do":

A. Where can I go to get more information on the new behavior I am considering starting?

B. What are the reasons I want to start this behavior?

C. What positive changes will occur when I start engaging in this behavior?

D. What small steps could I take to boost my confidence in this behavior?

I WILL DO

In the "I will do" phase, a person's level of inspiration and confidence has grown to a point where he is now beginning to prepare to change his behavior in the next few weeks. Usually there is a trip, a holiday, or a child's event that stands in his way of starting immediately, but as soon as that is over he is ready to go. It is best to strike while the iron's hot whenever possible. When you allow too much time to pass, you run the risk of dropping back to the "I might do" phase. People in the "I will do" phase have become more fully aware of the benefits and roadblocks of the behavior they are now ready to take on. With this awareness, it is wise to develop a structured plan to counter any setbacks, and to set S.M.A.R.T. goals.

As a trainer and coach, I don't always know if someone is being totally up-front with me. When I ask my clients how their diets are going, I usually hear the universal answer, "Great." What does that mean? "Great yummy" or "great healthy"? Probing and encouraging during this phase usually promotes the desired change because the perceived benefits are evident.

For months, Tanner, 39, told me he was ready to change his diet but just didn't have the willpower to do so. Because he believed that this was a weakness, Tanner's guilt continued to mount. Nine months into his training, Tanner reached the "I will do" phase with his diet. The pros in his decision-making process had increased to the point where he no longer could justify his guilt. Having two parents with heart disease and Type II diabetes outweighed his desire for ice cream, bread, and pasta. Within the next week, Tanner completely cut out all sugar and flour from his diet. With these changes, he noticed an immediate drop in his weight and triglyceride levels, and an increased level of energy.

CHAPTER QUESTIONS for "I Will Do":

A. What areas of my wellness are in the "I will do" phase?

B. Whom can I connect with to encourage and support me in my new behavior?

C. What challenges do I anticipate facing with this new behavior?

D. What are some "Plan B" ideas for when "Plan A" gets interrupted?

I AM DOING

This is the phase in which we have started a new behavior and continued it for just a few months. Since it hasn't become routine or we haven't seen the result we once envisioned, this new activity or behavior is at risk of stopping. If I sense that one of my clients is beginning to slip during this phase, I ask questions regarding the benefits of performing the new behavior and the consequences of not performing it. Also, helping clients not bite off more than they can chew is another way of promoting a slower change that will lead to a lasting change.

More often than not, people start their new behaviors too gung-ho! Burnout and the lack of a backup plan for challenging times usually end the new behavior. The following suggestions can help you increase the likelihood of continuing your new healthy behavior.

- Identify how your new behavior is influenced by what you value.

- Always prepare for a roadblock with an alternate plan.

- Regularly visit with your wellness coach about your behavior. (Note: a Certified Wellness Coach is one who is trained in how to work with people who are changing behaviors.)

- Have a wellness buddy or join a support group with similar goals, needs, and desires—people to go with you through these changes.

- Create a healthy environment in which you spend most of your time, an environment that strongly reinforces your behavior.

- Gain support from family, friends, and coworkers. These are the people who have the most influence over you and with whom you spend most of your time.

- Make a list of ALL of the benefits of your new behavior and the consequences of not performing your behavior, and post it where you will see it often.

There are basically two types of people I train at the gym: those who will perform workouts outside of our time together and carefully watch their food intake, and those who won't. It's easy to differentiate the two because one is more successful than the other. All of my successful clients have one thing in common: they all connect what they truly value with their fitness, health, and wellness S.M.A.R.T. goals. We all value something! Attaching that something to our goals and holding onto it makes the difference between being successful and not. It's that simple.

Brandon, 49, hit his stride in the "I am doing" phase when he began training with me a couple of months ago. The weeks leading up to his starting were spent contemplating the health changes he needed to make. Once he decided it was time, there was no turning back. Three months into his "new self," Brandon hasn't missed a workout with me or failed to do the home workouts he performs on his elliptical cross-trainer. He has cleaned up his diet to the tune of a twenty-pound weight loss and claims he has never felt better. A recent visit to the doctor confirmed the benefits of his efforts. Brandon's cholesterol, blood pressure, and blood sugar levels all reached desirable ranges.

CHAPTER QUESTIONS for "I Am Doing":

A. What is the BEST thing about my new behavior?

B. Who could be a continual support for me in my new behavior?

C. What changes to my environment can I implement to make it more conducive to my new behavior?

D. What will it take to maintain my new behavior?

I AM STILL DOING

This is the phase that we should all strive for in all areas of wellness. At this point, the behavior has become a habit because you have been fully engaged for several months. IT'S WHAT YOU DO! It becomes so ingrained in your daily, weekly, and monthly routine that it's uncomfortable to be out-of-rhythm with this behavior. Seldom do I see my clients quit their exercise programs to the point of losing all that they have gained once they have reached this phase. Most people will take a short break from their healthy behavior only to return to it quickly. In that instance, the loss of benefit is minimal. However, when people take a prolonged break, it is usually much more difficult for them to start back up. But, if they do, taking a closer look at what caused the break should help them make the necessary changes to prevent it from happening again.

Some helpful tips to stay in the "I am still doing" phase include:

- Know your alternate plan for any challenging situations that may arise.

- Become a role model and spokesperson to encourage people around you. Allow them to see your success, enthusiasm, and excitement. Coach and encourage others to consider doing what you have done.

- Try new and different healthy behaviors to prevent boredom.

- Continue to raise the bar on your goal-setting.

- Continue to seek support from family, friends, and coworkers of like mind.

- Keep your eyes focused on what is most important to you.

- Maintain the environment that has led to your success.

- Change your program from time to time to prevent plateaus.

- Stay current on health, fitness, and wellness information.

- Frequently remind yourself of your BEST-SELF VISION.

Taylor, 42, is the poster child for the "I am still doing" phase. She has what would appear to be the perfect life: a happy marriage with two kids, a habit of taking proper care of herself, and just enough balance with work and family life to keep everything running smoothly. Like clockwork, Taylor runs four days a week, five to eight miles a day; lifts weights twice a week; and attends yoga class twice a week. A healthy diet of meat, fish, eggs, fruits, and vegetables make up the bulk of her food intake. She has been in this phase for years and says she can't imagine doing anything different.

People like Taylor fall into the same routine that we all fall into: we get used to doing what we do and it becomes easy and comfortable to stay there, regardless of what the routine is. Taylor has two neighborhood friends who run with her regularly, and she employs me as her trainer. Even though Taylor might appear to be a hard-core fitness fanatic, she uses the social support and accountability of those around her to bolster her program.

CHAPTER QUESTIONS for "I Am Still Doing":

A. Where can I go to get more information on the topics of health, fitness, and wellness?

B. What other healthy behaviors would I like to try that generate the same results I'm looking for?

C. What will it take to stay focused on what is most important to me?

D. What support system do I currently have in place?

RESISTANCE TO CHANGE

Several years ago, I had one of those "ah-ha" moments during one of my coach-training classes with Wellcoaches when the instructor said, "People don't resist change; they resist being changed." For the longest time I struggled with not understanding why people fight changing their unhealthy, destructive behaviors. But this comment gave me new hope for working through this resistance in some of my clients.

As a result, I now take a new approach to my clients whose spouses react adversely to their nagging. Now I tell my clients to be patient and wait for their spouse to be ready to change. In the meantime, when appropriate, provide their spouse with the health consequences of his or her behavior. Here are a few examples of my clients and their situations:

1. **Sarah**, 49, constantly harps on **Cameron**, 56, to lose weight because she fears he will drop dead of a heart attack at any time. Knowing that her more aggressive "requests" have not worked in the past, she has now adopted a more subtle approach to get him to act. Sarah says things like, "Now, I'm not going to tell you not to drink those sodas anymore," or "You might not want to eat those chips." In addition, she frequently suggests that he go to the gym and exercise.

2. **Terah**, 43, rags on **Aiden**, 44, for his excessive drinking. She says that the drinking has contributed to his extreme weight gain and exacerbated his anger issues. Despite all of her complaints, Aiden still doesn't change his behavior. His attitude is "I feel fine, I don't need to quit drinking; I'll die when I die, and c'est la vie."

3. **Stacey**, 53, nitpicks **Ryan**, 57, for not exercising. She makes comments like, "If only you had been exercising, you wouldn't have injured your back," and "If you don't start exercising, you will have reoccurring back problems." These comments don't go over too well. Arguments always ensue. It's so bad that if

they hear an ad on the radio or television that has anything to do with exercise or back pain, all Stacey has to do is look at Ryan and he gets angry.

4. **Gary**, 68, expresses his displeasure with his sedentary wife **Jan**, 67, who constantly complains about being hurt, sick, or tired. He has grown so frustrated over the years with her whining about all of her infirmities that he lashes out at times almost uncontrollably. His "change what you're doing or stop complaining" approach only pushes her farther away from what she should be doing.

5. **Jeff**, 62, is disgusted by sixty-year-old **Kristen's** smoking habit before, during, and after her bout with breast cancer. She responds with a resentful comment anytime the topic of smoking comes up. Jeff can't say, "There's a new study that says smoking causes . . . " because it will be met with such strong opposition. She has been so successful in the other areas of her life, but she is reminded that this is her one true failure. Jeff has told me that her smoking has adversely affected their social life and sex life, has greatly reduced their level of intimacy, and led to their having both a smaller family and medical problems.

All of these naggees have one thing in common: they are all miles away from doing anything about their "condition." The naggers also share a commonality; they all believe they can force their partners into action by wanting them to change.

In all of these situations, no advice should be given unless it is solicited by the person who needs to change a behavior. The solution is to express empathy and communicate in a nonjudgmental, benign way.

Empathy feels good, real good. Anytime someone identifies with our feelings and our unmet needs we feel so much better. We're in a better position to change our behavior when we feel good about ourselves and we're not getting nagged. Recall a time when someone understood how *you* felt. How did that make you feel? Interestingly, your assessment of another's emotions doesn't even have to be correct; that person will still feel good just knowing that someone is in their corner.

As you engage in dialogue with someone, de-flaming the conversation is always a better approach. From the book, Being Me, Loving You: A Practical Guide to Extraordinary Relationships by Dr. Marshall B. Rosenberg, Nonviolent Communication (NVC) [2] seems to get people to consider other possibilities and to remove them from a conflicting, confrontational mode of communication. NVC is a lifelong practice. There are weekend retreats designed to help people strengthen their NVC and empathy muscles. The basic structure of NVC is:

1. *Make observations, not evaluations.* Anytime you judge someone, get ready for retaliation or isolation. Whatever the response, judging is not conducive to healthy, productive communication. Instead, reflecting back to someone what he or she just said helps the person know that you are listening, judgment-free.

2. *Differentiate feelings from thoughts.* These two are so often confused that most people don't even realize they are mixing them. For example, saying "I feel like you don't listen to me" confuses feelings and thoughts. This is very common in how most of us communicate. The words ". . . like you don't listen to me" don't describe a feeling. To separate the feeling from the thought, you might say, "I feel frustrated because you don't listen to me."

3. *Distinguish between needs and strategies to meet those needs.* "I need to go to the store" is another common but erroneous communication. Going to the store is a strategy to meet the need for eating.

4. *Make requests, not demands.* Little good happens when we demand something of another person. When we make requests such as "Would you be willing to . . . ," a softer response usually follows. And, in the request, you must include your readiness to hear "no" for an answer.

CHAPTER QUESTIONS:

1. What health-promoting change makes the most sense to me, right now?

2. What challenges do I anticipate encountering along the way?

3. How can I use empathy and NVC to better communicate with others?

CHAPTER 7
DEVELOPING A ROUTINE

Routines have the potential to create life or strip you of it.

What do you think of when you hear the word *routine*? Non-exciting, boring, same old thing, monotonous? Most people will probably tell you the same thing: routines are tedious, lifeless, and uninteresting.

What are your daily routines? Brushing your teeth after lunch each day, a shower at bedtime each night, coffee first thing in the morning? Whatever you do, you have a routine, whether life-giving, life-taking, or somewhere in between. Routines are huge, really huge! They can make life really easy or extremely difficult; they have a tendency to hold you accountable or captive; and they have the potential to create life or strip you of it. Depending upon the routine, relationships can be restored, health can be improved, and your work and life balanced.

Anxiety results when a life-giving habit is disrupted. For example, it is not uncommon for a triathlete to train for four hours or more a day. When this becomes the norm, everything takes a backseat to training. Many triathletes I know are often willing to sacrifice relationships, work, and important engagements, all for the sake of training. If they have to miss a training session, look out! They frequently feel anxious, guilty, and/or depressed because of this alteration in their routine.

Melissa, a forty-eight-year-old work-from-home wife and mother of two, illustrates this very point. With her husband still sleeping, Melissa runs five to eight miles every morning, Monday through Friday, at 5 a.m. Back home, she showers, prepares a healthy breakfast (such as eggs, bacon, and berries) for the family and sends them off to work and school. By 8:30 a.m., Melissa is ready to start her work day at home. During her lunch hour, she drives to the community swimming pool and swims anywhere from three-quarters of a mile to a mile and a quarter, depending upon how much time she has. Afterwards, Melissa returns home, grabs a quick bite to eat (usually leftovers from the night before), finishes her work for the day, prepares a healthy dinner of chicken, fish, or lean beef and vegetables for the family, and then goes to bed. On weekends, Melissa rides her bicycle twenty to fifty miles, when time permits. How's that for a life-giving, health-promoting routine? But, Melissa has not always been this driven with her diet and exercise program. She was able to parlay past successes from her work life into her self-care program and leverage those achievements to her advantage.

Routines that are not life-giving are often very difficult to change. Smoking, a sedentary lifestyle, and a poor diet are the most glaring examples of life-depleting habits. How many times have you or someone you know encountered extreme difficulty in smoking cessation, the "pain" of exercise, or frustration with nutritional misinformation? I hear about difficulties like these, throughout my work day, from people who are trying to change. It's tough, very tough! When you consider all of life's challenges, adding a major change to an already busy schedule can be daunting. But, here is the good news: Once you create these new, life-giving routines, the rest of your life becomes so much better.

Forty-three-year-old Bailey was stuck in a rut. His entire adult life had been spent consuming as many calories and expending as few calories as possible. A typical day consisted of going to work, where he sat all day, grabbing fast food for lunch, leaving by 5 or 6 p.m., going home, eating whatever was in the refrigerator or pantry, falling asleep on the couch watching television, then waking up and doing it all over again the next day. On average, Bailey went to the gym twice a week, when his friends could get him off the sofa. There, he lifted weights for forty-five minutes and walked on the treadmill for thirty minutes. According to his doctor, Bailey needed to lose fifty pounds and lower his cholesterol, blood sugar, and blood pressure. But Bailey's health issues are not pushing him to do anything more. He is content where he is in life.

When you make good decisions, good things happen, and when you make bad decisions, bad things happen, with a few exceptions. Whether it's exercise, smoking, stress, nutrition, or work/life balance, your habits today will greatly affect your habits and health tomorrow. In order to change habits, you have to seriously consider one or more of the factors that establish a routine:

- *Our Values* – Values are those things that are most important to us.

- *Our Spiritual Life Status* – Overall wellness is directly related to our spiritual life.

- *Our Stress Levels* – Stress tends to create a sense of urgency and may even stop us from acting.

- *Our Environment* – Those things that surround us every day often dictate our daily actions.

- *Our Beliefs* – What we believe to be true typically dictates our actions.

- *Our Comfort Level* – We often choose those things that are easy and comfortable.

- *Our Family and Friends* – The people closest to us often influence our actions.

- *Our Motivation* – What gets our attention gets us.

- *Our Profession* – The amount of time we spend working can't help but sway our routines.

- *Our Time Availability* – The routines we develop depend upon the amount of time we allot to them.

- *Our Dreams* – Following our dreams is a great way to establish health-promoting routines.

- *Our Level of Compassion* – How we feel about others determines how we spend our time.

- *Our Strengths/Abilities* – We tend to do the things we do best.

- *Our Attitudes and Thoughts* – What we think about our routines has a strong impact on our actions.

- *Our Level of Commitment* – Our general approach to commitment can either make or break a routine in the developmental stages.

- *Our Past Routines* – The ability to draw upon a positive past routine can increase the chance we will create new positive routines.

- *Our Current Level of Health, Fitness, and Wellness* – Positively or negatively, Newton's First Law of Motion sums it up perfectly: "An object in motion stays in motion until acted upon by an outside force . . . ."

CHAPTER QUESTIONS:

1. In what life-giving routines are you currently engaged?

2. How does it feel when you practice these routines?

3. What would it take to change some habits that are not life-giving?

4. How would your daily routine(s) then change?

CHAPTER 8

CREATING AN ENVIRONMENTALLY-SAFE WELLNESS PROGRAM!

Boredom and emotional eating are often opponents too formidable for willpower and good intentions.

I am blessed, really blessed, to work in a gym sixty-five hours a week. Granted, a sixty-five-hour workweek isn't the most enviable thing in the world, but the fact that I have absolutely no excuse not to work out is a really good thing. I have been told by many people over the years that it must be easy to work out every day because I "live" in a gym. I totally agree and that is one of the main reasons I chose to be a trainer: the environment in which I work is conducive to clean living.

But this isn't the case for most people. Several years ago, Stuart, 58, attended a two-week weight loss camp hoping to jump-start his need for radical change. He was given an eating plan and an exercise program, and took several classes on the various diseases that affect the overweight and obese population. Everything seemed to be working well until he returned home to face the "real world." With no game plan in place to address the emotions, stresses, and relationships in his world, he was doomed. Because Stuart was an emotional eater and always seemed to gravitate to comfort foods, he never had a chance to succeed with his new program. It left out one of the most important factors: how to deal with his environment.

We are victims of our own wills—healthy or unhealthy—and the environments we create around ourselves are products of our wills. The fact that we are driven by our desires and that we adapt to our environments can be a recipe for success or disaster. If we leave cakes, cookies, and candy in the pantry, we are more likely to eat them. If our home or worksite is not conducive to physical activity or has a high-stress atmosphere, we are likely to be sedentary and lead a stress-filled life. The people we spend time with, the restaurants we attend, the items we purchase at the grocery store, even the route we take to and from work all contribute to the success of our wellness plans. Changing any one of these environmental factors can have a dramatic effect on your plan's outcome. When my clients change their surroundings in a positive way, they greatly increase their chances of success.

Here are six common environmental factors you may need to change:

1. STRESS

What stressors do you have? Common stressors are work, relationships (marital, family, work, or social), community (local, state, or national), health, and finances.

We all know that whatever stressful situation you are experiencing, right now, has your full and undivided attention. However, other stressors, time passing, and stress reduction techniques have a way of diminishing the initial stressors hold on you.

What changes could you make to reduce your current stress level? Where could you go to learn more about stress management techniques to apply in your own environment?

Unfortunately, not all wellness stories have a happy ending. I had been training Pam and her daughter, Trisha, for the better part of Trisha's high school senior year. Over the summer, Trisha got very busy preparing to leave for college and her training stopped. That fall, everything was as it should be when you are eighteen and in college— AWESOME! Until it wasn't. Trisha and several of her friends were returning from a girls weekend several hours away when a pick-up truck hit them. Neither vehicle was traveling very fast, but Trisha—the only one not wearing her safety belt—was thrown from the car and died instantly.

Pam and her family were devastated. Pam became much more irregular with her workouts, and her stress level soared. As a result, her spiritual life took a big hit. She questioned everything she believed to be true about God. How could He have let something like this happen? A year and a half later, Pam was diagnosed with advanced breast cancer. She told me that her oncologist believed that it was the stress of Trisha's death that had led to her illness. After months of chemotherapy and radiation, Pam passed away. The continued stress not only stripped Pam of her health, but also eliminated her desire to seek healthy practices.

Would stress management techniques have helped save Pam's life? Could exercise and a healthy diet have eradicated the horrific physiological effects of her stress? What "environmental plan" could you put in place to help you deal with your stress?

2. NUTRITION/WEIGHT MANAGEMENT

What types of food do you purchase at the grocery store? Do you keep unhealthy food in your refrigerator or pantry?

Too often we lose the battle before we even start. Many people who are fighting to lose weight or to eat healthy, nutritious foods set themselves up for failure because of keeping unhealthy, non-nutritious foods in their homes. This can be devastating to our weight and our health. Carefully planning out what foods to eat and to keep in the house are powerful steps toward improving health and wellness.

Boredom and emotional eating can become obstacles too formidable for willpower and good intentions. Determine what healthy foods you want around you so that when you are "tempted" you won't have access to the foods that will harm you. Food is fuel, not therapy.

After sleep-walking for six months in the middle of the night to raid his roommate's food, twenty-six-year-old Jack finally put a lock on their refrigerator. This helped him get unstuck and lose the thirty-five pounds he had gained during those six months. Before his sleep-walking began, and during his day, Jack made good nutritional choices. Putting the lock on the refrigerator resulted in Jack's losing the thirty-five pounds as fast as he had put them on.

What foods need to be removed from your house? What healthy, nutritious foods should you add to your refrigerator and pantry?

3. EXERCISE

What is getting in the way of your regular exercise routine? Do you have access to a workout facility or exercise equipment?

This is a biggie because it is so easy to find excuses not to exercise, or worse, not to have an exercise program. Of all the areas of wellness, exercise is probably the most challenging for people to start and maintain with consistency. Therefore, it is imperative that you plan for success.

Joining a gym that is conveniently located; having a workout buddy; hiring a personal trainer or wellness coach for accountability; or having a walking/jogging partner can increase the likelihood you will both start and adhere to a program. You might purchase a treadmill or stationary bicycle for your home, or place your workout clothes in your car the night before you exercise—whatever it takes for you to create a better environment.

Thirty-four-year-old Amarie discovered early in her workout program that if she didn't work out at 5 a.m., it wasn't going to happen. The busyness of her job and her sheer exhaustion at the end of the day dictated the early morning exercise sessions. Amarie's success is generated by the environment that she creates for herself. The night before each workout she sets out both work and workout clothes and prepares her lunch for the following day. She always makes sure that she is in bed by 9 p.m. But, most importantly, Amarie chose to work out at a gym that is on her way to work, and to eat a healthy breakfast immediately following her workout, at a restaurant next to her gym.

How could you change your surroundings to accomplish your exercise goals? Where can you go to get more information on creating the right environment for your exercise program?

4. SLEEP

What is preventing you from getting the sleep you need? What habits could you change to get more high-quality sleep? What other areas in your life do you need to modify so they will help you?

With the normal hustle and bustle of work and family life, habitually high stress levels, large quantities of caffeine consumption, and our tendency to overextend ourselves, it's no wonder that our sleep patterns are adversely affected. Most people don't get enough sleep. Sleep interferences such as sleep apnea, restless leg syndrome, certain medications, and stress all contribute to the unhealthy toll that sleep deprivation places on our body. Studies have linked a lack of sleep to an increased risk of obesity, heart disease, diabetes, car accidents, and poor cognitive functioning. Additionally, a lack of sleep promotes bad decision making, especially with our wellness program. We are less likely to exercise when we are exhausted from sleep deprivation.

Payton, a sixty-two-year-old real estate developer, suffered from nighttime teeth-grinding. Until he went to his dentist and treated his grinding with a custom-fit, night mouth guard, neither he nor his wife got a good night's sleep. Once he began using his guard, both said they slept happily ever after. It's been several months now and Payton hasn't missed one night. He attributes his success not only to the desire to have healthy teeth and gums, but also to his surroundings: he places his guard next to his toothbrush so that he will put it in after brushing his teeth at night.

How many hours of sleep do you need to function at your best? What healthy lifestyle changes can you make to improve the quality and quantity of your sleep? What will it take to ensure that you will get that amount regularly? When was the last time you were caught up with your sleep? How did that feel?

5. WORK/LIFE BALANCE

Is your work environment conducive to building healthy routines? Most of us spend a large part of our lives working. If we don't discover ways to address our wellness at work, we will be fighting an uphill battle for our health. Finding ways to be active during your work day, practicing certain relaxation techniques throughout the day, and planning your lunch the night before will produce an environment where you are bound to succeed.

After watching a co-worker's health suffer greatly due to stress, thirty-four-year-old Malcolm decided to take matters into his own hands. After performing a few exercises in his office, he would complete a deep-breathing exercise, then take a five- to ten-minute work break, several times a day. Every time he did this routine, Malcolm said, it helped him get focused and centered. This refocusing created a more efficient and, for Malcolm, a shorter workday.

How can you address being overworked? What practices can you put in place to become more efficient at your work? What limits can you set during your day that would allow you to have more free time?

6. HEALTH/WELLNESS

How well are you? What areas of your wellness need the most attention?

When you evaluate your wellness, consider everything related to your emotional, physical, spiritual, and mental being. From happiness

to heart disease to fulfilling your spiritual needs to thinking clearly, this section discusses your entire wellness, not just the absence of disease.

Carefully design a plan of attack to address the areas you want to change right now. You must create an environment that will encourage success in each of these areas. Issues to be addressed may include:

- Planning doctor's appointments

- Planning family vacations and outings

- Regularly practicing stress management techniques

- Attending services to help you meet your spiritual needs

- Finding an exercise partner(s)

- Planning food intake several days in advance

- Spending quality time with loved ones to strengthen relationships

- Beginning counseling sessions with a licensed therapist

- Becoming more informed on health matters

- Employing a personal trainer

Staying on top of his health, thirty-three-year-old Hagan scheduled a doctor visit when he noticed a severe drop in his libido. Medical tests confirmed he had low testosterone. Because both Hagan and his wife wanted a second child, the doctor prescribed testosterone shots once a week. Creating an atmosphere of seeing a doctor when something's not right led Hagan and his wife to having their second baby boy several months ago.

What measures can you employ to improve your physical well-being? What steps can you put in place to help you grow spiritually, mentally, and emotionally?

In order to become alive and well, we need to pay more attention to stress level, nutrition and weight management habits, exercise and sleep habits, work/life balance, and current health status. You have the choice to design your life for success. How will you choose?

CHAPTER QUESTIONS:

1. What obstacles in your environment are preventing you from succeeding with your wellness program?

2. What will it take for you to raise your level of awareness about your environment?

3. What changes in your life need to be made to create a more health-conscious environment?

CHAPTER 9

FROM THE INSIDE OUT

Finally, I had an "ah-ha" moment:
an entirely new way of approaching
the drudgery of exercise.

Up to this point, we have looked at the meat and potatoes of establishing a wellness program and keeping it running. Now, let's turn our focus to several secondary factors that can positively affect your health and adherence to your self-care. Life's disappointments have a way of putting a damper on us. By strengthening the following areas in your life, you can greatly reduce the stress that often comes from not practicing mindfulness. You don't need to experience every one of these factors to create your program and life-long change; however, the more you do have, the greater your enjoyment and fulfillment in life.

We are in a constant struggle with a culture around us that encourages an attitude of "fight fire with fire." This outlook poses tremendous challenges. I hope that by drawing your attention to each of these factors, your awareness will be heightened to the point where you consciously choose to experience each one. Anything less and you are not living life to its fullest. The result of addressing each factor is an inherent boost in physical, emotional, spiritual, and mental health.

Although I do not expect people to focus solely on these, I certainly can testify to their health-promoting affects. Positivity just seems to flow from optimism. This chapter is full of "state of being" possibilities that will literally change your life if you put them into practice. Some of their life-giving benefits are:

- An overall sense of well-being

- Less stress and anxiety

- Less depression and negative thinking

- Lower blood pressure

- An improved immune system

- Reduced risk of cancer, heart disease, and other stress-related illnesses

- Better sleep

- Improved connections with other people

- Better relationships

- Greater life satisfaction

- Greater appreciation for life

- Greater longevity

- Greater coping mechanisms for illnesses and other life stressors

MINDFULNESS

Have you ever driven across town, reached your destination, and asked yourself, "How in the world did I get here? I can't remember driving to this place"? Or, have you ever gone back to check a door only to find you had locked it—you just couldn't recall having done so?

When I was twenty-nine years old, I was training for a marathon, running between 25 and 35 miles a week, lifting weights three hours a week, and eating a healthy diet. I decided to get my cholesterol checked to confirm my healthy lifestyle choices. Oops! The results showed a total cholesterol of 201 mg/dL, an HDL of 34 mg/dL, and an LDL of 133 mg/dL. The latter two were in heart attack range. How could this be? With all the time and energy I had put into taking care of myself, and while still young, I was at risk of a heart attack!

At about this time, several studies were published noting red wine's ability to raise HDL (good) cholesterol levels. I had been a non-drinking health fanatic, so those who knew me thought it a bit strange that I now took so eagerly to the bottle (or box, in my case). Eight months later, my HDL level had increased 50%, to 51 mg/dL. WOW! Before this, I had concluded that anyone drinking boxed wine was probably doing it for medicinal purposes only. I had no idea that wine could taste good or could be paired beautifully with food until my wife, Karen, and I went to a wine bar in Fredericksburg, Texas. It changed my life! I decided I had to learn more about wine and its production. Four months later, I was on a plane to Orlando, Florida, to take a two-day, first level sommelier course.

Both days began at 6:30 a.m. Once the instructors introduced themselves, we moved swiftly to lectures and wine tastings. The lectures focused on wine production all over the world and how wines differ from country to country and region to region. After each two-hour talk, we tested and assessed three wines. The first person in each group assessed the visual aspects of the wine, the second person the nose, the third person the palate, the fourth person the initial conclusions, and the fifth person gave the final conclusions on the type of varietal, the year, country, and region of the wine's production, and the name of the wine.

I studied each wine intently, whether it was my turn or not, and I found myself becoming more and more appreciative of each wine. The thought of whether or not I enjoyed the wine had never entered my mind. Now, I began to pay attention to all of the different things that wine could teach me. By eliminating all judgmental thoughts, I was able to focus on what I was experiencing "right here, right now!" As a result of this mindful practice, I came to appreciate wine on a whole new level. And I realized I could also apply those same attention-giving practices to whatever goes on around me in the present moment.

For the next several months, I tried to make my love of wine a part of my personal fitness training business. How about a group workout session followed by a wine tasting? Or wine parties where I invited only my clients? I was looking for that common thread that linked wine and exercise.

Finally, I had an "ah-ha" moment: an entirely new way of approaching the drudgery of exercise. I began teaching my clients who had negative thoughts and hang-ups about exercise how to assess what they were *experiencing* as they worked out. I had them address the following:

A. List three nonjudgmental adjectives (words or phrases) to describe what you are experiencing while you perform this exercise (an exercise that troubles you).

B. What do you notice throughout your body when you perform this exercise and immediately upon completion of the exercise?

I first tried this with forty-one-year-old Mollie. As one of my more vocal anti-love-to-exercise clients, Mollie never missed an opportunity to express exactly how she felt. Over the years before she became my client, the sweat, pain, and overall discomfort of the workout experience had gotten the best of Mollie to the point where her fitness was virtually non-existent. The fact that she was disease-free further suggested to her that everything was okay and that she could continue to eat what she wanted and not exercise. Mollie believed she was healthy.

An annual checkup at the doctor's office, however, indicated otherwise. Learning she was seventy-five pounds overweight and a borderline diabetic with high blood pressure and unhealthy cholesterol numbers led Mollie to me through a mutual friend. We met for a consultation, or fact-finding mission, as I like to call it, and Mollie described the source of her disgust with exercise.

She told me, "As a child, I was always made fun of for the way I ran, and as a result of that, I was also the last person chosen when it came time for picking teams. I wasn't very athletic at all."

"What does that have to do with your attitudes regarding exercise now?" I asked.

"I became so turned-off by doing any kind of physical activity that I would avoid it at all costs," Mollie said. "Any time a friend wanted to do something that required physical effort, I found excuses not to be available. Right now, years later, the very thought of exercise conjures up very unpleasant emotions."

I thought about it a minute and said, "What if you were to remove all of your judgmental thoughts from exercise? Do you think that might help?"

"I hope so," she said. "My health and maybe my life depend on it!"

At our first workout, I told Mollie my wine course analogy to help her understand the practice of mindfulness before she began working her abdominal muscles. When she completed her first set of abdominal crunches, I asked her what she felt.

"Pain, it made my abs hurt," she said. "I feel like I just got kicked in the gut."

"Okay." I said. "Do another set and remove ALL judgment from what you are experiencing."

After a second set she remarked, "It was difficult to stay that focused, but when I did I felt my abs shorten and lengthen and I noticed my breathing and heart rate increase." Mollie discovered that the more she practiced this mindfulness technique, the more she began to appreciate what she was experiencing while exercising.

If we could all look at our wellness in the same way we analyze wine, we would be much more aware of what is going on within ourselves. Wine became so much more when I paid attention to ALL that it had to offer (visual, nose, palate). This is true with life in general—the more you study it, the more you appreciate it, and the more wonderful it becomes.

It has been said that what gets your attention, gets you. When we are present in the moment and judgment-free, we are more likely to change our minds and our behaviors, and increase our control over healthy lifestyle decisions. This can be challenging at times, because we typically live our lives on autopilot. Frequently, we think about anything but what is going on right now. Mindfulness doesn't just happen. It has to be performed intentionally. Left to our own devices, we typically react to circumstances, often in a stressed manner, without taking the time to carefully analyze what the current situation has to teach us. This knee-jerk reaction only perpetuates itself.

But, as we become aware of the benefits of mindfulness, we become better able to handle stressful conditions and, therefore, are better equipped to make good, sound decisions. Unhealthy decisions might not be so popular if they generated instant repercussions. We can do things like eat a doughnut, miss a workout, smoke a cigarette, or bend over and pick something up incorrectly, without experiencing immediate consequences such as becoming obese, developing lung cancer, or herniating a disk, respectively. We tend to do these things because they are easier, faster, more comfortable, and make us feel better in the moment. What if you approached everything considering the consequences, first? You would drive your car defensively, always eat with good health in mind, and exercise with a purpose. This is what mindfulness looks like with your wellness.

Diet and exercise are of the utmost importance to me in regard to health and wellness. Unfortunately, these two areas often conjure up negative thoughts such as discomfort, dread, self-sacrifice, and self-denial. Thoughts like these are often the biggest roadblock most of us encounter. I face these thoughts on a daily basis with my clients. Negative thoughts are often the cause of a sedentary lifestyle among those who do not exercise regularly. But when you apply mindfulness to your diet and exercise, your habitual thoughts, both negative and positive, are removed and your appreciation grows. When we observe more and evaluate less, we eliminate the negative feelings and thoughts that have inhibited our workout programs in the past. You can eliminate negative feelings by finding nonjudgmental adjectives to describe what you are experiencing in the moment as you eat or exercise.

One thing I hear coaches say about their athletes as they improve is that the game begins to *slow* down for them. We tend to make mistakes when life goes too fast. When we take life's situations slower, we are better able to assess the circumstances in a clearer, more focused way. We are more likely to thoughtfully respond than have a knee-jerk reaction, resulting in an undesirable outcome.

This approach to mindfulness is what I call the **S.L.O.W.** (**S**ee what's going on around you, **L**inger over the situation, **O**perate your actions carefully, and **W**itness the results) method. It can help you become more mindful in life and, specifically, in your wellness program. The focus and attention required to self examine, generate new possibilities, set out a plan, and carry that plan out are instrumental to your program's long-term success. Consider the following examples of people using the **S.L.O.W.** method to create changes in their behavior.

Recently, I coached Susan, 56, on mindfulness. She said that her previous experience with mindfulness had created a greater willingness and desire to change her current exercise habits. Over the last couple of months, she had struggled to swim on a regular basis. Ironically, swimming was one of Susan's favorite activities. But with her job demanding more and more of her time, the inconvenience of driving to the pool, changing clothes, getting her hair wet, cleaning up, and then getting back to work seemed too overwhelming. Her motivation decreased as time passed.

Susan began with the **S.L.O.W.** model. She started to pay closer attention to every detail of what was going on with her body the few times she did swim on weekends. Her focus was on what she was feeling, emotionally and physically. She concentrated on the water hitting her body, as well as on each muscle contracting and every breath inhaled and exhaled. Her positive experience during swimming led to Susan's drastically changing her work schedule so that she could swim three days a week during her lunch hour. Her swim workouts became something that she wanted more of and that she had to have. She was dead-set on keeping her appointment with the pool. *Where there is a will, there is a way!*

I see it all the time in the gym: people just going through the motions of working out, thinking about everything but what they're doing. This creates a "have to" or "should" attitude towards their exercise programs. When you become more aware of your body's needs, limitations, and abilities, you are better able to appreciate your body's reactions to your workouts. Learning to stay focused on the task at hand involves using certain mind-body techniques.

I frequently remind my clients to focus on the primary muscle group that is working during a particular exercise. This, as studies indicate, generates a greater contraction in that muscle group and, subsequently, a more effective workout. Use this same mindful approach with any form of exercise. While you are exercising, ask yourself:

- What does my body need right now?

- What can I learn from this experience?

- Where is my body in space?

- What is my body feeling?

- How is my body benefiting from this workout?

As you continue to practice mindfulness during your workouts, you will notice increased body awareness at other times in your life. This, in turn, leads to a greater understanding of your body's needs.

Another example of how mindfulness can improve your wellness is with stress management. Stress leads you to hit a certain level of panic, due to negative perceptions. By removing all judgment, you remove the panic. Once you quiet the voices and noises inside your head, you are well on your way to reaching that judgment-free state. Ways to help you achieve this include activities such as listening to music, mowing the lawn, and taking a walk.

My client Richard, 57, experienced this very phenomenon. A prominent lawyer in our town, Richard's stress levels had reached epic proportions. With dangerously high blood pressure readings, one infection following another, and his doctor expressing more and more frustration with him, Richard decided he needed to cope better with stress. Once he began the **S.L.O.W.** method and listened to calming music, he became better equipped to handle that stress.

Richard also practiced becoming more mindful by writing down, in great detail, what all of his senses experienced as he observed a raisin (an exercise I had taught him in one of our coaching sessions). He answered such questions as: What color is the raisin? What is the raisin's shape? What does the raisin smell like? What does the raisin feel like in my hand and on my tongue? What does the raisin taste like? He became extremely focused and attentive using this exercise. When he applied this simple practice to other areas of his life, he found a much greater appreciation of those things around him. As a result, Richard lowered his stress level and its ill effects.

A third way mindfulness can assist you is through food intake. Identifying what you need and are feeling helps prevent mindless eating—eating for comfort, or out of boredom.

Brenda, 47, has battled poor food choices all her life. With her weight climbing, her blood pressure soaring, her energy level plummeting, and her doctor hounding her to lose weight, Brenda finally decided to make a change that greatly affected her life. She began to journal everything that she ate and drank throughout the day. She included everything she experienced then, such as the smell, color, texture, taste, and temperature of the food she was eating. She rated her level of hunger on a scale of 1 to 10 throughout her meal, paying very close attention to the difference she felt when the hunger number changed. Finally, Brenda described all of the emotions she felt from the start to the finish of each meal. She did all of this without judgment or evaluation. The more she savored and appreciated what she ate, the more balance she created in her eating patterns.

Brenda's mindful eating led her to:

- a much better grasp of what and how much she eats;

- a twenty-five-pound weight loss;

- lower blood pressure and lower triglyceride levels;

- a higher HDL (good cholesterol) level;

- a much more positive outlook on life; and

- a greater sense of well-being.

Finally, a fourth way in which mindfulness can assist you is in balancing your home life with your work life. Recently, I ran into Stephen, 46, a high school friend of mine. He had been burning the candle at both ends trying to get his new start-up company off the ground. Unfortunately, this meant Stephen was constantly on the go from the moment his feet hit the floor until his head hit the pillow. He hadn't spent any quality time with his wife and kids in months, he had not visited a doctor in years, he had not been exercising, he consumed a fast-food diet, and his stress was overwhelming. Stephen was in serious need of a work/life balance makeover.

I suggested a couple of mindfulness exercises, deep breathing, and a relaxation technique to slow down his mental chatter and help him get focused. A few weeks later, Stephen had made several schedule changes that allowed him to come home earlier two nights a week so he could spend more time with his family. Stephen told me that now when he felt stressed out, he practiced the deep breathing technique I had showed him and observed what he was feeling, physically and emotionally. When he practiced this throughout the day, he said, it helped him get focused and centered, again and again, to the end of his work day.

By removing judgment from your own self-examination, you are more likely to gain the confidence and appreciation you need to act on your desired changes. The following benefits of mindfulness can enhance your life.

1. Increased focus and attention

2. A new energy in moving forward

3. Less of the thoughtless, autopilot approach to life

4. New possibilities

5. Silenced judgmental voices of the past and future

6. Clarified thinking

When we consider our visions of who we want to be as a result of our wellness program, we are better served when we become more mindful and turn off our autopilot. By paying closer attention to everything that is going on around us, we are more likely to notice and appreciate the areas of our lives that need work. This is the point where self-talk is so important.

MINDFULNESS QUESTIONS:

A. How can being more mindful help you with your wellness plan?

B. What areas of your wellness need more attention and focus?

C. What questions might you need to ask yourself, when you are mindful, about your wellness (exercise, nutrition, weight management, stress management, work/life balance)? Here's an example, concerning nutrition. Before you eat something, ask yourself, "What are all the reasons I am eating this?"

GRATITUDE

As I reflect on the things for which I am most grateful, I am reminded of the many areas in which I am blessed: a beautiful and wonderful wife and three fantastic kids (all of whom are healthy), a great job as a personal trainer and wellness coach, terrific family and friends—my list goes on and on. To list everything would fill volumes, so I will just say, I am grateful for what I have. Gratitude is regarded as a virtue of the utmost importance for our overall well-being. It removes all entitlement. Whether we express gratitude or receive it, we have much to gain from its far-reaching health benefits.

When you approach every situation with an attitude that there is always something working, you are sure to enjoy the positivity that surrounds a grateful mindset. This, in turn, opens the door to a more positive outlook on life and an appreciative spirit. You can do this by giving thanks *in* and *for* all things. Research has shown that people who express gratitude are more likely to eat healthily, exercise regularly, have lower levels of stress, and experience fewer illnesses.

Mindfulness and gratitude go hand in hand. If we live life on autopilot, unaware of what is happening around us, our ability to appreciate and be grateful for things as they happen to and for us is obstructed. The more we notice the positive things in our lives, the more we are able to express and receive gratitude.

Inevitably, we all experience stress. Whether it is stress regarding your job, relationships, or illnesses, the ability to rise above the negativity that often accompanies stress rests solely on your capacity to be grateful in the moment. When stress hits, write out a list of specific things for which you are grateful in that situation. For instance, when a relationship gets challenging, make a list of those things that are good and are going well in the relationship. This will help steer you away from the negativity of stress-thinking. Whenever we are more positive, we are much better off emotionally, physically, and mentally, and we are more prone to act in healthy ways.

Have you ever known someone who never seems fazed by events that normally stress you out completely? Meet Brett, a thirty-six-year-old computer programmer. Married and with two young children, he understands his responsibility to be a good husband, father, and provider. Many of Brett's work projects require long hours and very technical knowledge. The time he needs to finish his projects is "never enough." Brett's calm, cool, and collected demeanor never ceases to amaze me. When faced with the heat of a deadline, he always comes through in time.

Brett is one of the most grateful people I know. In listening to him speak and watching his actions, I could tell he is thankful for all that he has. What's interesting is, I'm not sure Brett even realizes his grateful attitude has anything to do with his low-stress lifestyle.

The following ideas have helped some of my clients increase their experiences of gratitude.

1. *Journaling* – Writing down what you are grateful for every day lifts your spirit and improves your mood. This can be tough when things are not going well, but it can be done.

2. *Letter Writing* – Writing a thank-you letter to someone who has done something nice for you can be very therapeutic.

3. *Questioning Yourself* – By asking yourself, "What am I most grateful for?" you can immediately change your focus and mood.

4. *Focusing on the Positive* – I start all of my coaching sessions with, "What's the best thing that happened to you this week?" This gets people thinking positively and graciously. Also, it is common practice in my home at dinner time for each of my family to tell us the best thing that happened to him or her that day.

GRATITUDE QUESTIONS:

A. How could being more grateful improve your life?

B. What are you most grateful for?

C. What could you do to increase the level of gratitude in your life?

DISCIPLINE

Discipline is having control over the decisions you make. It is being able to accomplish a task regardless of your emotional condition. Stated another way, it is the desire to complete a task even when you don't want to do it at that moment. Discipline is more than finishing the last fifteen minutes of your workout when it is the most difficult; pushing that delicious dessert away because you know it is not in your best interest to eat it; or going to bed early to get the rest needed for a big day at work when your friends are urging you to spend time with them. No, discipline is doing all of these things *consistently*, regardless of how you are feeling.

Consider the following factors that influence your level of discipline. Rate each of these factors on a scale of 1 to 10 (with 10 the highest) in regards to an area of your life where you would like to have more discipline. For example, you want to start working out on a regular basis. Your commitment and willingness levels are at a 9, but your readiness level is at a 2. More than likely, you won't be disciplined enough to start, let alone maintain a program for any extended period of time.

> *Readiness* – How ready are you to start and/or maintain this new behavior? If your readiness level is low or lacking, it will be very difficult to start a new behavior. Determining how you can implement this new, healthy behavior in your schedule, and gathering as much information as you can about how this behavior will benefit you, will help increase your readiness level. Also, be sure to consider all of the negative health effects of *not* engaging in this new behavior.

> *Commitment* – How committed are you to this new behavior? The very nature of the word *commitment* requires getting something done when times are tough. Social support is a great way to increase your commitment level. Find friends or family members who will participate with you or provide you with the support you need as you embark on this healthy activity.

Willingness – How willing are you to start and/or maintain this new behavior? This is the most important factor. Bottom line: If you don't want to do it, you won't. The desire has to be there for any behavior to be performed over a period of time. When you identify the most important reason to take action and that reason evokes an emotional response, your willingness will grow exponentially to perform that new behavior. The most profound responses to the question of what's most important, typically occurs when you have hit rock-bottom or on cloud nine. When this reason is attached to S.M.A.R.T. goals that you have set, success follows.

DISCIPLINE QUESTIONS:

A. On a scale of 1–10, what is your readiness, commitment, and willingness to participate in an exercise program?

B. On a scale of 1–10, what is your readiness, commitment, and willingness to change to a healthier diet?

C. On a scale of 1–10, what is your readiness, commitment, and willingness to create balance in your work and home life?

D. On a scale of 1–10, what is your readiness, commitment, and willingness to be more proactive in managing your stress?

SELF-CONTROL

Self-control over weight and stress management, exercise, and work/ life balance is life-giving and health-promoting. Imagine having your weight right where you want it; your energy, strength, and endurance levels at an all-time high; a life where stress is easily managed; and complete control over your work life so that your life is "balanced" and your relationships are strong.

Recently, I was coaching Jessica, 41, about her nutrition. She admitted that she has absolutely no discipline when it comes to her diet. I have been trained to let the client come up with the answers for himself or herself. Midway through our conversation, Jessica brought up her need to say no. ALL of wellness comes down to ultimately one thing: SELF-CONTROL.

Generally speaking, choosing the unhealthy way in any area of your wellness is the easy way. So if your wellness program is to have any long-term chance at all, your level of self-control must be high enough to withstand the storms that your program will face. How effective would it have been if you were calm, cool, and collected during some of the more stressful times in your life? How might your health be better if you exercised more self-control at the dinner table? The list goes on and on—times when making good decisions would pay healthy dividends.

Self-control is nothing more than making good decisions. Unfortunately, it is a human tendency to do what we want to do rather than what we should do. That explains why such a small percentage of people exercise or eat right on a regular basis, or why when people do exercise or eat right, they do so for only a short period of time. Incorporating healthy behaviors into your lifestyle is challenging. However, the rewards extend far beyond the sacrifices made.

Here is a list of ways to help increase your self-control when you want to make healthy behaviors a lifelong endeavor:

- Weigh the pros and cons of a particular behavior. Not all pros and cons will carry the same weight. Evaluate each one so that you can make an accurate assessment. For example, one pro may outweigh five cons.

- Write out the "right" thing to do, not the easy thing.

- Set S.M.A.R.T. goals and have another person hold you accountable for the goals that you set.

- Write out a list of the benefits and consequences of the healthy behavior you are considering. Make sure to include feelings associated with both.

- No matter what, get it done. Perform the healthy behavior consistently. Become so informed about your behavior (for example, by reading about health research and reading books by well respected authors) that you know exactly why you are doing what you are doing.

- Write down what you experience with your behavior; how it makes you feel; what you are learning from the experience; what your biggest obstacles are; and the strategies you can use to overcome your obstacles.

SELF-CONTROL QUESTIONS:

A. How could increasing your self-control affect your wellness?

B. What areas of your wellness need more self-control?

C. What can you do to increase self-control in those areas?

LAUGHING

Laughter's positive effects are a big boost to our overall wellness. Driving to work one day, I saw a marquee that read: "If you can't laugh, it's going to be a long day." How true is that? Laughing is one of those things that makes life worth living. Personally, I love to laugh. It improves my mood, attitude and is fun. Laughing acts as a wonderful escape from some of life's many stresses and creates a bond with other people around me.

Research tells us that laughter is good for our physical, emotional, and relationship health. By spending time with those who make you laugh, watching funny movies, or smiling at yourself in the mirror, you improve your well-being.

LAUGHING QUESTIONS:

A. How often do you laugh?

B. How could your wellness be improved by laughter?

C. What can you do to laugh more?

FORGIVENESS

When we forgive others, we reduce the stress-inducing conditions that lead to heart disease, ulcers, cancers, and countless other ailments. When we are happy, we recover from illnesses faster and have lower blood pressure, a stronger immune system, and a stronger heart and arteries. Clearly, our physical health improves as other areas of life improve.

So, how do we forgive the man who walks into McDonald's and guns down several innocent people eating dinner; the molesters of our children; the drunk driver who kills our loved one; or the person who spreads rumors about us? At some point, we are all faced with resentment, anger, and bitterness. But these emotions only tear you apart and lead to greater stress in your life. The persons you are angry with, or resent, might not even be aware of your feelings, and chances are they don't care.

So why forgive? It's just so easy to hold a grudge. Plus, if you don't, you're letting the other guy off the hook, right?

However, when you decide to forgive someone, you let go of all of the negative, stress-inducing feelings that are holding *you* captive—the kind of stress that leads to illness. When you forgive someone, you are not saying that what they did was right; you are untying the grip it has on YOU. Focus on all of the positive benefits that can come from this experience. Once you have done this, you will be on your way to a much healthier life. Practicing forgiveness on "small" issues will prepare you for the larger ones and will help boost your forgiveness confidence.

FORGIVENESS QUESTIONS:

A. What are your attitudes towards forgiveness?

B. Whom do you need to forgive?

C. How might forgiveness improve your health?

FAITH AND HOPE

According to Hebrews 11:1, faith is believing in what you long for and trusting in the unseen, regardless of your circumstances. Assurance and hope go a long way toward explaining how we react to and internalize life around us. As belief and trust in something grows, so does our faith in it. For example, people who place their faith in God tend to follow the tenets of scripture as seen in Galatians 5: 22-23. Typically, they display more hope, peace, faithfulness, joy, grace, mercy, forgiveness, love, and other godly traits.

Frequently, faith is viewed in Biblical terms, where faith and obedience go hand in hand. Regardless of where we are spiritually, we are constantly exercising faith. We place our faith in a chair to hold us up, a car to get us across town, and family and friends to have our best interests at heart. We must have faith in the behavior that we are considering for it to take hold in our lives. Once that faith is evident, our compliance to that behavior is more likely than without that faith. Consequently, when that faith weakens, adherence to our healthy behavior diminishes as well.

When we do not see the fruits of our wellness labor or we are disease-free in spite of neglecting our health, it is easy to lose faith in what is best for us. Most of the time exercise makes us feel better, but that does not always mean that we will see the weight loss or strength increases that we hope to see. There are so many benefits to exercise, seen and unseen, all the way down to the cellular level. It can be easy to lose sight of some of those unseen benefits. I see many of my clients become content with limiting their exercise to the one to three hours a week that they spend working out with me. They do not believe that any additional exercise will have any positive effect on their health because they do not feel sick.

To increase your faith, learn as much as you can about the object that requires your faith. The object must deserve your faith or you won't invest in it. Once you have done this, slowly put into practice ways to establish that faith. For example, it's highly unlikely that some-one would eat a healthy diet who lacked the necessary faith that it would produce positive results. So, if you fall into this category, learn as much as you can regarding the benefits of proper nutrition. Once you have read enough information to convince you, slowly replace "bad" foods with "good" foods and observe, over time, what you are expe-riencing. Consider your energy level, body weight, blood cholesterol, and blood sugar levels. What other changes do you notice? As you see the positive changes grow, so will your faith in your program.

FAITH QUESTIONS:

A. What area(s) of your life could be improved by increasing your faith?

B. Where in your overall wellness would having more faith have the most profound effect?

C. What could you do today to increase your faith?

HOPE

Hope is the belief in a realistic outcome that produces a desirable result. Hope says, "There is *always* a better way. Your future good health resulting from the positive changes you make today will be so much better than your 'poor' health created from your past." It has an ongoing presence in our lives in most things that we experience; but it isn't until we're tested that we realize our level of hope. For example, we often take our jobs, families, and health for granted. It's not until one of those things is threatened that we start displaying our desire and need for it. Our hope is strengthened when we discover our life's meaning and purpose, connect with similar past experiences that have led to success, and realize that there has got to be a way out of our predicament.

When was the last time you heard an inspiring story, one that really struck a chord with you and tugged on you emotionally? How did it make you feel? That feeling is hope welling up inside of you. It increases your determination and strengthens your will. Hope creates an energy and excitement about future possibilities as it pushes and drives you to a better future and to a higher level of performance. Hope always has a positive outlook and approaches situations with an "I can" or "It will" attitude. Hope feels good, which leads to an increased readiness to start a new behavior. It keeps us fighting for a desired outcome when all appears bleak. It pushes us to be our best. Hope generates passion and purpose and produces persistence and determination regarding our wellness. It gives us a reason to get up in the morning.

Having no hope has devastating effects and is usually a symptom of larger life issues. Imagine living a life of despair, despondency, and gloom. The end result is spiritual death and often a physical death, too. If you feel this way, you should seek the help of a professional counselor.

HOPE QUESTIONS:

A. What area of your life needs more hope?

B. How can hope lead to an improvement in your health?

C. What steps can you take to improve your level of hope?

GRACE AND MERCY

I can't mention grace without mercy and vice versa. Both are similar but very different in nature. *Grace* is unmerited favor, getting what we do not deserve. It is more about being, rather than doing. Grace is loving another person in his or her imperfection and forgiving that person regardless of his or her actions and whether or not he or she asks for forgiveness.

So what does grace have to do with wellness? The transfer of grace is one of the more powerful ways of expressing love and, therefore, reducing your stress. When we give grace, we communicate love to another person; when we receive grace, we allow the other person the joy of loving us, and the benefits are far-reaching. Grace calms your spirit. It is energizing and gives life meaning and purpose. Grace produces happiness and improves our life satisfaction. It strokes our soul and creates unconditional love. The list goes on and on!

GRACE QUESTIONS:

A. To whom can you extend grace today?

B. How will you extend that grace?

C. How could grace improve your health?

Mercy, on the other hand, is not getting what we deserve; it is a release from judgment. It is a two-way street: to receive mercy, you must render it to others. Alexander Pope, an eighteenth-century English poet, said, "Teach me to feel another's woe, to hide the fault I see; that mercy I to others show, that mercy show to me." [1]

If mercy is rooted in love, kindness, and gentleness, its backbone is compassion. Mercy helps those in need or in distress. By its very nature, it means performing good works for other people. It stands to reason that when we receive mercy our well-being is enhanced; but, what happens when we extend mercy to others?

These good works reduce stress and improve immune function. They lead to a decrease in illnesses and an increase in longevity. Good works can also create in the giver a sense of purpose and meaning in life. When these good works are performed, the hormone oxytocin is produced, which creates a feeling like a runner's high. Good works feel good.

MERCY QUESTIONS:

A. To whom do you need to show mercy?

B. What feelings will you be able to discard by showing that mercy?

C. How might mercy improve your health?

KINDNESS/GOODNESS/GENTLENESS

Research shows that even fake-it-till-you-make-it kindness has health benefits for the giver, receiver, and those who witness it. Acts of kindness stimulate the release of serotonin, which produces a euphoric feeling, and makes us feel good about ourselves. When we feel good about ourselves, we are more likely to act in healthy ways. Kindness is ultimately an issue of the heart, from which all behaviors are born. The positive feelings generated by kindness acts have a way of moving us to take other actions.

By learning the benefits of doing certain healthy activities and the consequences of unhealthy behaviors, we are in a better place to start and maintain a self-care program. We are strongly influenced by our emotions. Wouldn't it be better to be driven to action by our positive emotions rather than our negative ones? That is not to say that because we are kind people we are automatically going to practice regular self-care. What it does mean, though, is that our hearts are in the right place to make a change and to do so for the right reasons.

KINDNESS QUESTIONS:

A. What was the last act of kindness you performed?

B. How did that make you feel?

C. In what ways did it improve your health?

PEACE

Perhaps peace makes you think about a quiet, still, serene place with calming, soft music. This may include a glass of wine and a hot bubble bath, and perhaps no children within sight or sound. Perhaps the lighting is low and the atmosphere is very relaxing. Sounds peace-producing, right?

Wrong. I'm not talking about that kind of peace. Authentic peace is being in the middle of life's stresses and troubles and having a stillness of heart, mind, and soul. It has nothing to do with our circumstances but everything to do with the condition of our spirit. When we address life's challenging circumstances with a positive mindset and a spirit of what's working best in our lives, we grow our authentic peace.

Practicing many of the additional factors that I have discussed in this chapter will help produce an authentic peace.

- Loving and forgiving others
- Practicing gratitude and charity regularly
- Extending mercy and grace whenever possible
- Growing spiritually
- Increasing your faith and hope
- Practicing kindness

PEACE QUESTIONS:

A. How much peace do you have in your life?

B. What could you do to get more?

C. How might that affect your health?

LOVE

In the Greek language there are three forms of love, *phileo* (friendship), *eros* (romantic), and *agape* (unconditional). Agape is the backbone. All three types of love serve our well-being as we practice them regularly. Several years ago I came across a definition of love that has stuck with me: *Love is humility in service and self-sacrifice.* So far, this definition has never failed me. It exemplifies the very nature of the word and has a place in all relationships.

What effect does love have on our well-being? Well, in addition to connection, intimacy, interdependence, and sense of purpose—great health!

Because love is a choice, the more you give to and the more you do for others, the more love you will have for them. The more you focus on the goodness of others, the more your love for them will grow.

LOVE QUESTIONS:

A. Whom in your life do you love with a *phileo* love? *Eros* love? *Agape* love?

B. How do you demonstrate that love?

C. What could you do to increase that love?

D. How do you see love affecting your health?

E. What can you do to love the "difficult to love" people in your life?

JOY/HAPPINESS

What makes you happy? Is it having wealth, being disease-free, or receiving that promotion you always wanted? We are constantly being told through advertisements in the media that we will be happier if we buy their products, use their services, or look like their models. Research, however, indicates otherwise.

At some point in time, we have all looked for happiness in all the wrong places. "If only I had more of this or less of that, I would be happy," we might say. Studies show that we can be happy regardless of our circumstances. What does any of this have to do with our wellness? Well, happy people are more cautious about their health, deal with pain better, have lower blood pressure, and are more likely to do something about their well-being. As a result, they will be more successful with their wellness programs. Plus, who doesn't want to be happy?

JOY QUESTIONS:

A. What activities bring you the most joy/happiness in life?

B. How does that joy/happiness influence your willingness to do something healthy?

C. What changes can you make today to be happier?

D. How does happiness influence your overall sense of well-being?

TRUTH AND HONESTY

"Honesty is the best policy" is definitely true when dealing with yourself and others. Truth matters. I am not referring to our individual perceptions of truth. I mean truth in the form of honesty, and its relationship to our overall well-being. When you choose to be ignorant to avoid unwelcomed news regarding your wellness, you deny yourself the universal need for honesty. You can't afford not to know the truth about your health and your relationships.

In Chapter 6, I referred to Nonviolent Communication (NVC) as the most effective way to express empathy. Empathy is the respectful understanding of another person's experience. Expressing empathy is done by identifying the needs and feelings of other people. By strengthening your honesty muscles, you will increase the connection and trust you have with other people and deepen your relationships.

This all sounds great, doesn't it? Well it is, but it's not always easy. At some point you have to have "THAT" conversation. Do you ever go along to get along? Do you choose the path of least resistance in your relationships? It's easy to do, but more often than not, there are consequences to those decisions. By keeping certain conversations to yourself, you miss out on the intimacy and connection that gives life to relationships. When honesty becomes commonplace in your relationships, stress levels plummet. And stress is the root of so many illnesses.

TRUTH AND HONESTY QUESTIONS:

A. Do you feel connected to those closest to you?

B. Are you honest with the people in your life?

C. How important is honesty to you in a relationship?

D. Recall a time when honesty was at an all-time high in one of your relationships. How did that feel?

E. How do you think that honesty has affected your health?

COMPASSION

I recall a time, several years ago, when I arrived home after a long work day. With rush-hour traffic, the workday's usual stresses, and my normal daily fatigue, I had had it! My mood was not inviting. I sat on the couch to decompress. Before I knew it, my youngest daughter, Lauren, had snuggled up next to me. She didn't say a word; she didn't have to. Her compassion spoke volumes. She knew that I had had a really hard day. It meant so much! Her presence let me know that whatever I was experiencing she was "in it" with me. That is what compassion does; it reassures us that we are not alone no matter how bad things get, and it seeks to alleviate the suffering of another person.

Just as in practicing all of the other factors, when we practice compassion, our souls are at ease and our inner turmoil is alleviated. As you grow in all of these areas, not only will your relationships thank you, but so will your well-being.

COMPASSION QUESTIONS:

A. How do you show compassion to those around you?

B. How would practicing compassion on a regular basis improve your stress levels?

C. How would it improve your relationships?

D. Recall a time when someone was compassionate with you.

E. How did it feel?

F. How did it enrich your life?

CHARITY

There is no better way to fight the stress war than to do it through charity. When we act charitably, we give our lives purpose and direction, as well as enrich the lives of others around us. "No good deed goes unpunished" is incorrect. All selfless acts pay dividends regardless of how they are received. I prefer the statement "Virtue is its own reward."

By nature, we are self-centered beings. When we act benevolently and seek first to meet the needs of others, not only do others benefit, but we become happier as a result. The happier we are, the more likely we are to engage in healthy behaviors. Giving to others has been shown to reduce stress, anxiety, and depression. In helping others, you step outside of yourself and focus on them. When our attention is on the needs of others, our moods and attitudes quickly become more positive. Who doesn't want more of that?

By helping others selflessly we can improve the lives of everyone involved. Charity has such a profound effect on us that we benefit even when we are not directly participating in it. The greater the sacrifice, the greater the reward.

CHARITY QUESTIONS:

A. What are some ways you can become more charitable?

B. How could your health benefit from giving your time, talents, and treasures?

C. What feelings would you experience by becoming more charitable?

PATIENCE

When we over-expect results, our healthy behavior under-delivers. This can be frustrating, considering we live in a "hurry up, right here, right now" society. Consider the recent college graduate who expects a six-figure income, the hundreds of thousands of people who regularly purchase lottery tickets hoping to strike it rich, and the patient who takes a pill expecting an immediate cure. They all have what our culture has impatiently come to expect: an unrealistic acquisition of success. Unfortunately, this mindset can lead to disappointing setbacks that interfere with future efforts toward positive behaviors.

A greater understanding of what to expect and when is important to help keep healthy behaviors from becoming former behaviors. To increase our patience, we must encounter situations that require us to exercise patience; it's a trial and correction approach. The things that lead us to feel frustrated, irritated, and aggravated are the same things that will strengthen our patience. Over time, our patience muscles grow and get stronger as we correct the trials of our experiences.

With elevated gas prices and a need to increase my patience, I have taken on the task of driving really slow. By slow, I mean no faster than 45 to 50 mph and with a very slow and gradual acceleration from stoplights and stop signs. Initially, I did it to save gas, which it has. However, driving slow has also bolstered my patience. Obviously, the tendency is to drive faster and avoid the honking and hand gestures that the other drivers feel compelled to express. This is the point where my patience grows.

As our patience grows, we become better equipped to handle the obstacles that our self-care will inevitably encounter. This, in turn, strengthens our persistence and adherence to our program. With adherence comes greater confidence and lasting change.

PATIENCE QUESTIONS:

A. What can you do to strengthen your "patience muscles?"

B. What area of your wellness needs more patience?

C. How could exercising more patience help you with your overall wellness?

POSITIVE THINKING

All of the factors that I have discussed up to this point culminate in positive thinking. If nothing else, through positive thinking we benefit from all the other factors and have a more optimistic outlook.

I am reminded of the story of the Two Wolves (the source of this story is unclear). One evening a grandfather told his grandson about a battle that goes on inside people. He said, "My son, the battle is between two wolves inside us all. One is Evil. It is anger, envy, jealousy, sorrow, regret, greed, arrogance, self-pity, guilt, resentment, inferiority, lies, false pride, superiority, and ego. The other is Good. It is joy, peace, love, hope, serenity, humility, kindness, benevolence, empathy, generosity, truth, compassion, and faith." The grandson thought about it for a minute and then asked his grandfather, "Which wolf wins?" The grandfather replied simply, "The one you feed."

If we allow negative feelings to dominate our thoughts, they will generate catastrophic stress levels. Who wants to spend time with others who are angry, jealous, greedy, arrogant, and resentful? Negative feelings can destroy relationships with your spouse, family members, friends, colleagues, and neighbors. On the other hand, by centering your life on practicing *forgiveness, happiness* and *compassion,* in addition to *faith, hope,* and *love,* you reduce stress, enrich your relationships, improve your overall sense of well-being, and increase your life expectancy. Bottom line: You will feel fantastic!

I continuously encounter the negativity people have towards diet, exercise, and wellness: I don't have enough time; this is too hard; I'm not losing enough weight; I can't lift this much; and countless other comments when things get tough. This negativity paralyzes any forward movement to create a better future. Positive self-talk loosens negativity's grip. With a positive outlook, we alleviate stress, irresponsible eating, a lack of desire to exercise, and a whole host of other negative health behaviors. People with a more positive outlook take better care of themselves and are more successful with their wellness programs.

By becoming more mindful of the sources that produce our negativity, we generate more appreciation and positive feelings toward our problems. When you engage in an interest that is more important to you, the problem conducting the negativity loses its energy and hold on you. This leads you in new directions and to new possibilities.

If we learn to appreciate our struggles, we can learn and grow from our experiences. I remember one of my wellness coach instructors telling our class that the optimist says, "The glass is half-full"; the pessimist says, "The glass is half-empty"; the appreciative person looks at the glass and says, "My, what a beautiful glass." Just imagine the changes possible in your life when you approach your wellness with that attitude. Capturing all your negative thoughts and replacing them with positive ones leads to endless possibilities.

POSITIVE THINKING QUESTIONS:

A. "Which wolf wins" inside of you?

B. What areas of your life do you tend to be negative about?

C. How could positive self-talk affect your health?

CHAPTER 10

THE ZONE VS. DISRUPTION

Seeking the zone on a daily basis is critical to any wellness practice.

The old adage that says we do things that will bring us pleasure or prevent pain should be my gym's mantra. When we are denying an area of our wellness, it is usually because we are giving something else our time and attention. We seek whatever is most comfortable. At first glance, "whatever is most comfortable" appears to be universal, meaning everybody's idea of comfort is the same. But, if that were true, we would all rather lie around, eat and drink whatever we wanted, sit rather than stand, and drive instead of walk. For a good number of people that is true, hence the weight and health epidemic our country faces. But people who practice a healthy lifestyle on a regular basis have often found themselves in the zone with their wellness program, and they seek it again and again.

You know you have hit the zone when your level of success equals the challenge at hand. You are able to match the energy and intensity that the activity in which you are engaged requires. It almost seems effortless at times. Each successful moment rolls over into the next phase of your skill. You are at the top of your game and performing at your highest possible level. A high level of self-confidence, skill difficulty, and desire each play a major role in entering the zone.

Disruption happens any time we are performing a task and we are not in the zone. Things just don't seem to fall into place. Alison, age 47 and weight 330 pounds, really tried hard to enjoy her workouts. But any form of exercise was truly drudgery to her. She scheduled only one workout a week with me and cancelled at least twice a month; this behavior did not allow her the opportunity to develop any kind of rhythm.

As a personal trainer, I am probably the most lied-to person on the planet. Alison's diet was atrocious, but if I were to believe Alison, she wrote the book on how to starve herself. She never admitted to eating anything because she was so embarrassed and, most importantly, not ready to change. She didn't want any guilt about or correction to her eating habits. This too is an example of a disruption on Allison's path to good health.

Unfortunately, our world is made up of people with lives disrupted directly by their health. Jesse, age 65, had gained about 75 pounds. During the years in which he had gained that weight, his body had deteriorated; he now had no energy and it hurt to move. He'd had joint replacement surgery in his late fifties. Jesse's blood sugar and triglyceride levels were dangerously high. He was not in a good place physically. I would like to tell you that he got in the zone, and everything worked out beautifully. But I can't. I lost track of Jesse years ago. I hope he made the necessary changes to turn his life around.

I am not an expert skier, and I ski only every ten years or so. I start the week on the bunny slope only to end the week on a more challenging black slope. From snow-plow to downhill, parallel skiing. Not only does my confidence grow, but so does my ability to perform the skills needed to successfully maneuver down the mountain without killing myself. When my confidence is high and all is "clicking" and I am "in the groove," I am in the zone.

Your wellness program needs to be in the zone for you to carry it out for any significant period of time. Remember, the zone and your level of comfort do not mean easy. Being in the zone simply means your self-doubt is low and your ability high. Since we typically like to do things we are good at, choose activities at which you are proficient and that you enjoy. You are more likely to stick with those practices for the long haul. By applying this guideline to your exercise, food intake, work/life balance, and stress management, you set the stage to reap "ginormous" benefits. Seeking the zone on a daily basis is critical to any wellness practice that you perceive at first as uncomfortable or undesirable.

All of this will be demonstrated when you develop a routine. Living a healthy lifestyle in the form of a regularly scheduled, well thought out, daily, weekly, monthly, and yearly plan is mastering the ideal of becoming your best.

Adam, 56, is an insurance salesman who travels constantly. He spends one or two nights at his home during the week, and on the weekends he often visits his father, three hours away. Somehow, Adam always finds time to exercise early in the morning, three to four days a week. When he returns home from his weekend trip, he sets his menu for the week and grocery shops so that he is fully prepared. Every September, Adam schedules his doctor appointments for January so that he sees his internist, dentist, and ophthalmologist for that year.

Denise, 52, loves her yoga class three times a week. She is also an avid runner and runs four miles, four or five times a week. If she is traveling and has to miss running, she always makes it up. Fortunately, she usually travels to a city where she is familiar with the running tracks near her hotel and can fit in her four miles without a problem. Like Adam, Denise is very regimented about her diet and she plans it out carefully. Both Adam and Denise have told me that once in a blue moon they treat themselves to an alcoholic drink or dessert. They share one thing in common: they are both in the zone with their routines, and the routines work! They both believe that if they take care of themselves now, it will be much easier and cheaper later in life.

CHAPTER QUESTIONS:

1. Recall a time when you were in the zone in one of your wellness areas (exercise, food intake, stress management, etc.).
    What were you doing?

2. How did it feel?

3. What can you do to get in the zone in all your areas of wellness?

CHAPTER 11
CARPE DIEM

. . . when confidence is high, success follows.

Motivation is one of my favorite wellness topics because there is so much mystery behind it, and it forces me to connect with what is most meaningful to me. What comes to mind when you think about what you value most in life? Do you think about God, family, friends, and health? What else comes to mind? How do those values relate to your wellness, health, and fitness levels? What motivates one person toward self-care doesn't always motivate another person. This is because of differences in what each person values. I cannot tell you the number of times a client has said, "I'm just not motivated to workout or change my diet." What I hear is, "I haven't attached what is most important to me to goals that I set for myself," or "I probably need to set some goals." Therein lies the key to motivation: keeping your attention focused on what you value most.

I believe there is greatness in all of us; it is just a matter of tapping into the perfect combination of motivation, determination, persistence, resilience, and confidence. I hope this book has struck a chord within you and is motivating you to reach that greatness. Not everyone will be an astronaut, the CEO of a large company, or a professional athlete, but we all have the potential to do the extraordinary when all the parts are in place.

Meryl, a fifty-nine-year-old housewife, is one of my more interesting clients. I began training her in 1996 when she decided she wanted to improve her fitness level and lose weight. As she began to lose weight, she realized that what she really wanted was to improve her self-image. It has been this desire that has kept her on track with her wellness program for the last seventeen years.

Thirteen years ago, Meryl was diagnosed with breast cancer. Throughout chemotherapy and radiation, she never missed a beat with her workouts and weight-loss program. I have seen the opposite before: people often give up their healthy practices and let the medical world take over. Not Meryl. She became more positive and optimistic about her future. This created more drive and inspiration to keep on keepin' on. There was no feeling sorry for herself. Meryl molded her 160-pound body into a sleek 135-pound frame over the course of our training. More importantly, she has KEPT THOSE POUNDS OFF!

So, what kept Meryl motivated before, during, and after her diagnosis? How she viewed herself became the focal point of her motivation and her ability to face one day at a time. Each day she did all she could possibly do to make it the best day ever. Never did she dwell on the negative.

What's most important to you? What is your focal point for keeping your drive alive? The best way to measure your motivation is to look at the actions you are willing to take to reach your goals.

So many times I hear about or see people who start their programs strong only to fade over time. What's the secret to keeping the motivation at a high level even when you are connected to what you value? Nothing kills motivation like unrealistic expectations. When S.M.A.R.T. goals are not the foundation of your plan, feelings associated with defeat often set in. For example, the "goal" of losing a certain amount of weight by spring break or summer becomes entirely too daunting a task when you have incorrectly written your goals. The following reasons may strip your desire to continue working at a level high enough to reach your desired change:

- Realizing the large amount of work required to accomplish the "goal";

- Thinking the results don't happen fast enough;

- The physical "uncomfortableness" of the process;

- The time required and inconvenience created, generally; and

- The inconvenience created with work, family, and other engagements.

By setting S.M.A.R.T. (specific, measureable, action-based, realistic, and timely) goals, you put yourself in a great position to stay motivated and succeed. Also, participating in activities that you enjoy and at a time and place that work best for you go a long way towards helping you stick with your program.

When you understand the meaning and purpose for which you are performing an activity and develop a certain level of proficiency at it, you are more likely to continue the healthy behavior. For example, regular exercise provides purpose in the form of better health, more energy, and a greater sense of well-being for most people. When this realization is combined with a high skill level of a particular activity, desire to perform the task follows. When this happens we become highly motivated.

Another important ingredient in staying motivated is confidence level. Think back to a time when you successfully completed a task. You probably felt good about yourself and your ability to complete that task. Success at a given activity is the driving force behind the belief that you can perform that same task the next time you try. I see it at my gym all the time: when confidence is high, success follows. Why is that? Are we thinking things into existence? No! The higher our confidence level, the greater our effort. There is nothing we won't try if we believe we can do it.

Over the years, many of my personal training clients have told me when they were starting a new diet or adding more exercise to their workouts at home. They were in search of a quick fix to whatever health issue affecting them. Regardless of the diet or exercise program, every one of my clients had one thing in common; they all believed that they would be successful because someone they knew was successful with it. Identifying with another person's success that is close to you can have an enormous affect on your drive and motivation.

Two men were camping in the woods when they noticed a bear charging towards them. One of the men sat down and started putting on his running shoes. The second man asked, "You don't actually think you can out-run that bear, do you?" The first man replied, "Of course not, all I have to do is out-run you!"

What motivates you? Looking and feeling your best, having more energy, or overall better health? Have you ever started a diet, workout, or wellness program, only to see it crash and burn despite all of your well-intentioned efforts? Ask yourself these questions:

1. What makes this (the task you want to perform)
   really important to me?

2. Is this answer strong enough to get me past any
   obstacles I may encounter?

3. What 'bear' in my life is chasing me?

SUCCESS BREEDS SUCCESS

Success is doing what you should do, not what you could do—doing the next right thing. In other words, doing that which feeds the soul and is life-giving. The more we seek to do those things we believe we should do, the more successful we feel; the more successful we feel, the better we feel about ourselves; the better we feel about ourselves, the more effort we are willing to exert. This can have a domino effect in all areas of our lives.

Mother Teresa is a wonderful example of doing what she believed she should do. By caring for the rejected, poor, and sick, she fulfilled the "should do" deep inside her spirit. According to letters she wrote, she experienced a sense of abandonment from God throughout her selfless service. This provided a great opportunity for her to say "I could do" something else. But, as we all know, Mother Teresa opted to remain in the ministry, living out her service. How's THAT for success? Sainthood!

Let's bring this down to a level where you and I can apply it to our lives from a wellness point of view. Think of a time when you were successful and your confidence was sky-high. How did you feel? What steps did you take that led to your success? How can you transfer the important elements of that situation to your fitness program, nutrition, sleep habits, stress management, and work/life balance?

I was eagerly awaiting my son's first tackle-football scrimmage. Aside from being one of the three biggest players on the team, he had the dubious honor of being the youngest by six months. Some of his teammates were three years older and had experience playing football. David's challenge was to learn fast and develop at ultra-speed. Prior to the scrimmage, David had been relegated to second-string on both the offensive and defensive lines. Taking this all in stride, David had not complained about his position on the team.

For the scrimmage, the coach had moved David to the first-string, right offensive tackle. I thought if David were to have any success in football, it would be on the offensive side. After all, being the "All-Pro" armchair quarterback that I am, I have all the answers. Later in the scrimmage, David got his shot at defensive tackle. Wow! David ended up with two tackles and forced two fumbles, one of which he recovered. The coaches slapped David's helmet and shoulder pads, and cheered and praised him for his efforts. For the rest of the scrimmage, he jumped up and down between each play, and encouraged his teammates to pick up their play.

When we got home, David re-enacted everything that had happened for the rest of our family. From that point on he became ÜBER-BOY! Anyone who has tried to get an eight-year-old (especially a boy) to do his nighttime routine knows it is like pulling teeth to get him to do any of it. Now, David took a shower and actually washed his hair. After he ate dinner, he took his dishes to the sink and rinsed them off before putting them in the dishwasher. He brushed his teeth and came to show me he was doing a good job. All of this without being asked. Then he said, "Come on Dad, it's time for me to go to bed." WOW!

Success breeds success. With success and praise comes extreme effort. Even the most mundane things in life can be appreciated and completed with energy and enthusiasm. And with increased confidence comes the desire to motivate others.

CHAPTER QUESTIONS:

1. What are your primary motivators for engaging in healthy behaviors?

2. What causes you to lose motivation?

3. What could you do to prevent that from happening?

CHAPTER 12
FREQUENTLY ASKED QUESTIONS

When insulin levels rise,
fat is stored in your body's fat cells.

Q: *How do I make my overall wellness program something I WANT to do rather than something I HAVE to do?*

A: The quick answer is, simply engage in healthy life-giving activities that you enjoy. The more social you make the activity, the more likely you will take pleasure in it and the more accountable you will become. Another way to "WANT" to participate in an otherwise uncomfortable activity is to set easy-to-reach S.M.A.R.T. goals to help increase your confidence and motivation. For example, if you enjoy walking, a S.M.A.R.T. goal might be to walk on Monday, Wednesday, and Friday for ten minutes at 8:00 a.m. If you do this long enough, your success will lead to increased motivation and more challenging goals. You'll be more inclined to do things with a positive attitude when you see progress. Most people who stop healthy activities do so because of unrealistic expectations and low motivation.

Q: *I was sore for two days after my last workout. Is that normal?*

A: Soreness, or delayed onset muscle soreness (DOMS), is a result of unaccustomed exercise. Training is very specific and your body will adapt to the stimuli that you give it. It is common for soreness to result from a workout, especially if you haven't worked out in a while. Also, changing your workout can lead to soreness if the new workout is more intense than your usual workout. DOMS is thought to result from microscopic tears in the muscle fibers exercised. The amount of damage depends on the duration and intensity of the exercise. Usually, soreness begins to subside in a couple of days as muscle fibers repair and rebuild themselves, leading to an increase in strength and endurance. Ways to treat DOMS include light stretching, rest and recovery, active recovery (low intensity) at the end of a workout, massage, taking a non-steroidal anti-inflammatory drug, and eliminating inflammatory foods such as, vegetable oils.

Q: *I am exercising several times a week but still not losing weight. What am I doing wrong?*

A: Most likely it is your diet. When you exercise, your appetite increases; that is why it's so important that you eat to compensate for that in a healthy way. Eating foods high in carbohydrates, especially easily digestible, processed carbohydrates, leads to water retention and elevated insulin levels. These foods contain sugar and processed flour. When insulin levels rise, fat is stored in your body's fat cells. When insulin levels remain low, fat is mobilized and used for energy; it is burned off.

Q: *How do I flatten my stomach?*

A: You reduce the amount of fat between your abdominal muscles and your skin. This is done by developing the muscles in the abdominal area, by aerobic exercise, and by a diet that reduces fat. Unfortunately, there are no exercises that will directly reduce the fat in your abdominal area, an approach called spot reduction. By exercising your abdominal muscles with crunches and other core exercises, you develop the muscles under the layers of fat that will show when the fat is reduced. A diet low in carbohydrates will help reduce the circumference of your waist by mobilizing fat stores and using the fat as fuel.

Q: *I find myself grazing from the time I get home from work to the time I go to bed. How do I get this under control?*

A: There are several reasons why this happens:

1. You didn't eat enough earlier in the day, and you're famished by the time you get home.

2. You're bored.

3. Your eating becomes mindless.

4. Your emotions dictate your desire for food.

5. You're eating a lot of non-satisfying, easily digestible, high carbohydrate foods.

The responses to these causes are self-explanatory: eat more throughout the day; engage in an activity at night that demands your full attention; become more mindful, especially when you are eating; limit your eating when you are emotional; and eliminate the easily digestible, high-carbohydrate processed foods from your diet. More often than not, these solutions are easier said than done. However, by asking yourself, "What do I need, right now?", being more present in the moment, and attaching your values to S.M.A.R.T. goals, you are better equipped to make good decisions and succeed.

Q: *My motivation seems to start strong and then quickly fade. How can I keep my motivation at a high level to eat right, exercise, and get the sleep I need?*

A: Nothing kills motivation like unrealistic expectations. When S.M.A.R.T. goals are not set, the feelings associated with defeat often set in. I see this with New Year's resolutions; the "goal" of losing a certain amount of weight by spring break or summer becomes too daunting a task. Remember that the following reasons typically strip your desire to continue working at a level high enough to reach your desired change:

- Realizing the large amount of work required to lose the weight;

- Feeling results don't happen fast enough;

- The physical "uncomfortableness" of the process;

- The time required and inconvenience created, generally; and

- The inconvenience created with work, family, and other engagements.

By setting S.M.A.R.T. (specific, measureable, action-based, realistic, and timely) goals, you put yourself in a great position to succeed and stay motivated. Participating in activities that you enjoy and at a time and place that work best for you go a long way in helping you stick with your program. When you understand the purpose for which you are performing the activity and develop a certain level of proficiency at it, you are more likely to continue the healthy behavior.

Q: *Is 20 to 30 minutes of exercise two or three times a week enough exercise?*

A: Most professional organizations claim that 20 to 30 minutes of exercise on most days of the week is enough to improve your cardiorespiratory health. However, including the necessary resistance, aerobic, and flexibility training will take longer than that. I have found that a good rule of thumb is five hours a week. In that amount of time, you can spend two or three hours a week resistance training and two or three hours in aerobic and flexibility training.

Q: *With my schedule, I am always on the run. As a result, my diet suffers big time! Convenience is of the utmost importance! How can I get control over what I am eating?*

A: The combination of ease and convenience in easily digestible, high carbohydrate and processed foods, and the hustle and bustle of the American lifestyle, are not conducive to eating a healthy diet. It has been my experience that planning a healthy, nutritious diet on a weekly or monthly basis is the best approach. This allows you to make a good decision when you encounter a time crunch and when other obstacles get in the way.

CHAPTER 13

STRATEGIES FOR GETTING STARTED

Strike while the iron's hot.

I remember walking to and from school every day, playing kickball and bombardment in P.E. class, playing football and basketball every day after school with the neighbors, and riding my bicycle up and down my neighborhood's hills. It's easy to take for granted those days when others were "overseeing" your exercise. Whether you are accountable to yourself or to another person, success often hinges on your reporting your progress to someone.

My clients rely on me, as a personal trainer and wellness coach, to hold them accountable. If I have learned one thing in the twenty years I have trained people, it is that the majority won't maintain their workout/dietary program without someone there to hold them accountable. My clients say, "I didn't want to come today, but I knew you were here waiting for me," or "I didn't want to be charged for this workout and not show up." Whatever the reason, accountability holds your feet to the fire and helps you stay the course when motivation is running low.

UNCOMMON MOTIVATION STORIES

I am a big proponent of doing whatever it takes to get and stay motivated. Here are a couple of unique examples of how some people stay motivated.

Motivation Story #1

Several years ago a fellow personal fitness trainer, Dan, trained Carlos, 38, who needed an interesting tactic to get motivated. Weighing in at 300 pounds when they started training, Carlos was able to lose 120 pounds in the first year and a half of their training. Having come from a military family, Carlos needed to know that he was tough, but that his trainer was tougher. About once a week, and less frequently as the years passed, Carlos pushed Dan's limits. This only happened when they were the last two people in the studio for the night. When he was told to perform a particular exercise, he would refuse to the point where Dan began hitting and pinching him. This was a test to see if Carlos could resist Dan's "attacks." This always led to an all-out wrestling match in the center of the fitness studio. This reassured Carlos of the hard work he had been doing to lose weight. Carlos only defended himself; he was never the aggressor. After each bout, Carlos regained his mental toughness until the next time it "needed" to happen.

Motivation Story #2

One of my longtime clients, Connie, 34, began waking up at 4:00 a.m. to walk on the treadmill for an hour before her day started. Before she got on the treadmill, Connie went into her bathroom and put on her bikini. After several minutes of evaluating her physique in the mirror, she quickly put on her workout clothes and jumped on the treadmill. It was a constant reminder of what she wanted to leave behind.

Motivation Story #3

Alex, a thirty-year-old account executive, uses *mindful exercise* techniques to help him avoid his negative thoughts and feelings about exercising. Without these techniques, it is virtually impossible to get him "excited" about exercise. With the techniques, he better manages his utter disdain for fitness. When Alex focuses consistently during a few workouts on what he is experiencing while exercising, free of judgment, his appreciation for exercise grows. This leads to a greater desire to train and to more challenging workouts. When Alex's focus is lost, it is like pulling teeth to get him to do anything of benefit. This same process plays itself out with his food intake.

Motivational Story #4

I love tough people. In Chapter 1, you met Margaret, age 89—the toughest person I have ever trained. In the two years Margaret has trained with me, she has never whined or complained about anything. Several months ago, Margaret was hospitalized for three weeks with the flu. Her hospitalization fell within a ten-week period in which Margaret had other health problems that kept her from working out, too. A bout with the flu can be tough on anyone, but Margaret is blind in one eye, uses a walker, and survived polio 84 years ago, leaving her with a nonfunctioning left leg. She also suffers from dementia. A week after her hospital discharge, Margaret, wearing slippers and with disheveled hair, was back in the gym ready to work out. You can imagine how weak she was after the flu and three weeks of bed rest. Margaret was so weak that she couldn't get up on her own from the benches and machines where I placed her for each exercise; yet, she still worked out. Fortunately, there was a trained caregiver in the gym who lent a hand to Margaret's son and me as we got Margaret up and "running" again.

As I was assisting Margaret on one of her exercises, her husband, Arthur, who had been walking on the treadmill, shouted out, "Rusty, turn the heater on. It's too cold in here."

I had the air conditioning and fans running because the gym would have been burning hot had I turned them off.

Margaret, who is very soft-spoken, said to me, as she threw her hands in the air, "I'm so tired of hearing him whine about everything."

The following list will help you stay connected and engaged in the changes you expect to make. The more of these you put into practice, the greater your chance for success.

STRATEGIES

1. *Make a Commitment* – Making a commitment to yourself or another person enhances the chance of your success. Thinking "I'll try" won't work. That phrase is the ultimate bailout because you always have an out, an excuse not to succeed.

2. *Design a Plan* – Having a plan of action, a vision, gives you direction and a sense of focus.

3. *Create a Social Support System* – Joining a group of like-minded people increases adherence to and accountability for the new, challenging healthy behaviors.

4. *Contact and Hire a Specialist to Get Started (Wellness Coach, Personal Trainer, Nutritionist, Massage Therapist, and Preventative-Care Doctor)* – Speaking to people in the preventative healthcare business is not only a good idea but a necessity. These professionals can help steer you in the right direction.

5. *Accountability Buddy* – Having an accountability buddy increases responsibility and motivation.

6. *Start a Wellness/Gratitude Journal* – Writing in a journal keeps you connected to your healthy behaviors.

7. *Gather Information* – Accumulating information regarding health and wellness helps you make good, sound, and educated decisions.

8. *Strike While the Iron's Hot* – Start your new routine when your energy is at its highest. Act on your excitement as soon as you can; it will bolster your motivation.

9. *Brainstorm* – Generating ideas of those wellness activities that are most compelling to you will help give you initial direction.

10. *Assess Your Needs* – Measuring what you need will give you additional insight into your overall program when it comes time to design your S.M.A.R.T. goals.

When you commit to giving an account of your program's goals, you increase the probability of succeeding. Exercising any one of these strategies will help you develop a solid, sound approach, especially when motivation is low.

Just as Michael had experienced after his incredible loss of 200 pounds in eleven months, Ava, 33, had "it," then lost "it," and is now trying to find "it" again. Trying to regain the desire to practice a healthy lifestyle can be quite arduous once it's lost. Ava started out with a bang, quickly changing her diet and exercise. Within the first couple of weeks we worked together, Ava created a wellness journal that she wrote in every day. She wrote down everything she ate, all of the exercise that she performed, and graded her stress levels daily. This continued for about a year. Then she changed jobs at about the same time her father-in-law passed away, and her self-care eroded quickly.

A year later, Ava still has not hit her wellness stride. She just can't seem to manufacture the drive she had when her motivation led her to a twenty-pound weight loss, significant drops in her blood glucose and LDL cholesterol levels with an increase in her HDL "good" cholesterol, and, by her own admission, plummeting stress levels. Unfortunately, she has regained the twenty pounds plus about ten more and developed chronic low-back pain that greatly affects her activity level. All this ultimately led to depression, killing any desire to rev up her willingness to take care of herself.

My hope for Ava, and others like her, is that she will find that certain something that will jump-start her motivation again. Because we tend to act according to the state of our emotions, getting "right" emotionally is the key. Having a more positive outlook can propel us into a lifetime of wellness and self-care.

How is your outlook on life? What can you do to make it more positive? The answers to these questions could determine how and when you start and stay with your wellness plan.

CHAPTER QUESTIONS:

1. Who is holding you accountable for your wellness program?

2. Which strategies are most compelling to you?

3. How many strategies do you think you must use to be successful?

BENEFITS AND SUGGESTIONS

Always consult a physician before starting any exercise program, a registered dietician or nutritionist before any nutrition program, and an exercise professional for an exercise program prescription to best fit your individual needs.

The Institute of Medicine recommends one hour of vigorous exercise every day to maintain cardiovascular health, body composition, and ideal body weight. One hour a day may appear unrealistic for many people with busy schedules. It should also be noted that many studies indicate that twenty to thirty minutes a day of moderate exercise will provide cardiovascular health benefits.

Use one the following formulas to determine your Target Heart Rate zone when performing aerobic exercise.

1. Non-Resting Heart Rate (RHR) Formula

220 - Your Age = Predicted Heart Rate Maximum (PHRM)

PHRM x 60% (.6) = Lowest end of the heart rate zone

PHRM x 85% (.85) = Highest end of the heart rate zone

Example: A 20-year-old female wants to train in her target heart rate zone (60-85% of PHRM):

$$220 - 20 = 200 \text{ (PHRM)}$$

$$200 \times .6 = 120 \text{ bpm}$$

$$200 \times .85 = 170 \text{ bpm}$$

Therefore, this 20-year-old would want to train at an intensity of 120 - 170 bpm, her Target Heart Rate (THR) zone.

---

2. RHR Formula

$$220 - \text{Your Age} = \text{PHRM}$$

$$\text{PHRM} - \text{RHR} = \text{Heart Rate Reserve (HRR)}$$

$$(\text{HRR} \times \text{Training \%}) + \text{RHR} = \text{THR}$$

Example: A 50-year-old male with a resting heart rate of 65 bpm wants to train at 70% of his PHRM. (bpm = beats per minute).

$$220 - 50 = 170 \text{ bpm (PHRM)}$$

$$170 - 65 = 105 \text{ bpm (HRR)}$$

$$(105 \times 0.7) + 65 = 139 \text{ bpm}$$

Note: A true RHR is taken when you wake up, before you get out of bed.

EXERCISE
Benefits:

- Helps perform daily activities with greater ease

- Improves mood

- Increases energy

- Improves sleep

- Improves sex life

- Improves athletic, work, and recreational performance

- Reduces the risk of some cancers

- Strengthens muscles, bones, and joints

- Lowers blood pressure

- Lowers the risk of heart disease, stroke, osteoporosis, and osteoarthritis

- Increases the level of good (HDL) cholesterol

- Lowers the risk of diabetes

- Increases flexibility

- Increases lean body mass

- Lowers triglyceride levels

- Reduces the adverse effects of stress

- Makes new brain cells, which aids in learning

- Can generate an endorphin high

- Reduces back pain

- Improves body image and self-confidence

- Boosts the immune system

- Reduces risk of premature death

- Helps control weight

- Improves balance and body control, reducing falls

- Improves memory

- Strengthens the cardiovascular and respiratory systems

- Improves self-esteem

- Enhances sense of well-being

Suggestions:

- Walking

- Running

- Swimming

- Cycling

- Stationary-Bike Riding

- Elliptical Cross-Trainer

- Tennis

- Racquetball

- Basketball

- Resistance Training

- Yoga

- Pilates

- Bootcamp

- Zumba Dance

- Exercise Toning Classes

Note: Exercise is any activity that overloads and improves the cardio-respiratory and/or musculoskeletal systems. Certain activities do not overload these systems adequately and are therefore not considered exercise. Overload is experiencing any exercise resistance greater than what is encountered on a regular daily basis.

PROPER NUTRITION AND HYDRATION
Benefits:

- Weight loss/management

- Increases energy

- Prevents/treats diseases (Type II diabetes, cancer, heart disease)

- Helps protect brain function

- Helps with muscle and bone development

- Positively effects how you look and feel

- Improves cellular health

- Lowers blood pressure

- Improves sleep

- Supports immune function

- Improves focus and attention

- Enables proper fetal and childhood development

- Improves self-esteem

- Creates a greater sense of well-being

Suggestions:

- Consult with a nutritionist.

- Read as much information as you can, from reliable sources, regarding diet and nutrition.

STRESS MANAGEMENT
Benefits:

- Reduces blood pressure

- Decreases the risk of heart attack and stroke

- Reduces the effect of free radicals on cells

- Reduces anxiety

- Improves immune function

- Increases peace of mind

- Improves sleep

- Improves relationships

- Creates greater emotional stability

- Creates a greater sense of well-being

Suggestions:

- Develop your daily prayer life.

- Get more sleep.

- Exercise regularly.

- Eat a healthy diet.

- Reduce alcohol intake.

- Write in a wellness journal.

- Engage in thoughts and activities that help you outgrow your stress.

- Do something you enjoy.

- Take a hot bath.

- Get a massage.

- Listen to calming music.

- Read a book.

- Learn to forgive.

- Avoid superfluous stress.

- Establish techniques on how to cope with your stress.

- Use deep breathing techniques.

- Create a stress-free environment.

SLEEP

Benefits:

- Increases energy

- Improves mood

- Improves memory

- Reduces the risk of developing Type II diabetes

- Increases longevity

- Improves focus and attention

- Enhances creativity

- Creates a greater sense of well-being

Suggestions:

- Research indicates that 60–70°F is the optimum temperature for quality sleep.

- Keep your room as dark as possible.

- Reduce wine and caffeine consumption prior to sleep.

- Exercise regularly.

- Go to bed and wake up at the same time every night and morning.

- Read a book at bedtime.

- Listen to soft music at bedtime.

- Avoid eating just before bedtime.

- Take a warm bath or shower just before bedtime.

- Turn off the television and computer at bedtime.

WORK-LIFE BALANCE
Benefits:

- Improves relationships with family and friends

- Reduces stress associated with work

- Increases rest time

- Decreases risk of work burnout

- Increases time for exercise and recreational activities

- Enhances sense of well-being

Suggestions:

- Develop a daily prayer life

- Learn to say no at work

- Don't take your work home with you

- Get more active in community activities

- Eliminate unnecessary, energy-draining activities from your life

- Exercise regularly

- Find more time for relaxation

- Be who you are, where you are: a spouse and/or parent at home, and an employee at work

- Have regular date nights with your spouse

- Regularly schedule "me" time into your schedule

- Limit overtime work and reduce business travel, when possible

WEIGHT MANAGEMENT
Benefits:

- Prevents obesity and obesity-related illnesses (heart disease, stroke, Type II diabetes, cancer, obstructive sleep apnea, high blood pressure)

- Makes you look and feel better

- Maintains energy levels

- Reduces the number of body aches and pains, especially back pain

- Maintains sex drive and sexual satisfaction

- Prevents musculoskeletal strain

- Maintains the ability to perform normal daily activities

- Maintains self-confidence

- Enhances sense of well-being

Suggestions:

- Exercise regularly

- Do not eat or eat sparingly those foods that will cause you to gain weight

- Know your metabolism

- Drink plenty of water throughout the day

- Write in a food journal

- Find a friend who is into weight management, work on it together

- Get adequate amounts of sleep

- Manage stress levels

ACKNOWLEDGMENTS

My relationship with Christ is at the heart of my wellness journey. I grew up in a Christian home, attending weekly church services and annual Christian retreats. Although I had called myself a Christian for the first twenty-two years of my life, it wasn't until my senior year in college that I accepted the gifts and promises that my Father was offering me. I owe my parents everything for introducing me to Truth while I lived under their roof. It made all the difference and has directed me to over-achieve in this life.

I am deeply indebted to all of my clients, who have not only taught me so much, but who have also tolerated my endless conversations about this book's topics. Those conversations have generated many thoughts and led to greater insights into people's health behaviors. I appreciate Rocky Wilcox for helping me connect with the Texas Medical Association and Andy Weary for his letter of recommendation. Thanks to Mike Coffin and Patrick Nolan, I have a fantastic website, book cover and journal design. I am grateful to Catherine MacDermott, Laurie Drummond, and Suzanne Batchelor for taking the time to edit the book and raise it to a much higher level. I am very thankful for Wellcoaches, whose coach training helped me find more ways to help people in the area of wellness. I owe so much to my wife Karen, and my children Brittany, Lauren, and David, for their patience and encouragement throughout this entire process.

Most of all, I am grateful to my heavenly Father for creating in me the desire to help others and to use this medium as well as my personal training and wellness coaching business to do so.

ABOUT THE AUTHOR

Rusty Gregory is coauthoring *Living Wheat-Free For Dummies* (Wiley Publishing) set to be published in February, 2014. He received his B.S. (Commercial and Industrial Fitness) in 1989 from Texas Tech University and his M.S. (Kinesiology) in 1991 from the University of Michigan. In 1991, he began his personal training business in Austin, Texas, and became a Certified Strength and Conditioning Specialist (CSCS) with the National Strength and Conditioning Association (NSCA). In 1995, he opened Forte Personal Fitness, a personal training studio available to personal trainers and their clients. Rusty became a Certified Cancer Exercise Specialist with the Cancer Exercise Training Institute when he saw the particular needs that cancer patients have before, during, and after diagnosis and treatment. He is a Contributing Expert for dailyRx.com.

Rusty is also a Certified Wellness Coach (CWC), a Wellcoaches certification. He helps people make lasting behavioral changes that lead them to become their best selves. Coaching has allowed him to become more empathetic with people and their wellness "issues." He has seen many realize a higher level of wellness and begin to live life with more depth, meaning, and purpose.

In writing this book, Rusty drew upon his experiences as a personal fitness trainer and wellness coach as well as his formal training and certification in both fields of study. His extensive academic background has influenced the writing of this book and given him the tools to train people in a way that enhances their lives through health, fitness, and wellness. To learn more about health, fitness, and wellness visit his website www.RustyGregory.com.

Rusty lives in Austin, Texas, with his wife and three children.

For Rusty, Kent M. Keith's Paradoxical Commandments* say it all:

1. People are illogical, unreasonable, and self-centered. Love them anyway.

2. If you do good, people will accuse you of selfish ulterior motives. Do good anyway.

3. If you are successful, you win false friends and true enemies. Succeed anyway.

4. The good you do today will be forgotten tomorrow. Do good anyway.

5. Honesty and frankness make you vulnerable. Be honest and frank anyway.

6. The biggest men with the biggest ideas can be shot down by the smallest men with the smallest minds. Think big anyway.

7. People favor underdogs, but follow only top dogs. Fight for a few underdogs anyway.

8. What you spend years building may be destroyed overnight. Build anyway.

9. People really need help but may attack you if you do help them. Help people anyway.

10. Give the world the best you have and you'll get kicked in the teeth. Give the world the best you have anyway.

*The Paradoxical Commandments were written by Kent M. Keith as part of the second chapter of his booklet, The Silent Revolution: Dynamic Leadership in the Student Council, published by Harvard Student Agencies in 1968.

ENDNOTES

CHAPTER 5

1. Epictetus. Concerning such as read and dispute ostentatiously, Chapter xxiii. Retrieved from http://www.bartleby.com/100/715.html

2. Margaret Moore and Bob Tschannen-Moran, *Coaching Psychology Manual*, (Philadelphia: Lippincott, Williams, and Wilkins, 2009).

3. G. T. Doran, "There's a S.M.A.R.T. way to write management's goals and objectives," Management Review, Volume 70, Issue 11 (AMA Forum), 1981, pp. 35–36.

4. Bob Tschannen-Moran, "Provision: #496: SMART GOALS," Life Trek, Inc. d/b/a Life Trek Coaching International. Retrieved from http://www.lifetrekcoaching.com/provisions/20070121.htm "LifeTrek Provisions, an acclaimed inspirational e-newsletter, published weekly by LifeTrek Coaching International (www.LifeTrekCoaching.com) – a professional life coaching, career counseling, and organizational development company – is delivered to some 15,000 people in 152 countries. School Provisions, an e-newsletter published by the affiliated Center for School Transformation (www.SchoolTransformation.com), applies coaching principles to enhance educational leadership and school environments. We encourage you to sign up for either or both publications."

5. William Penn (1644–1718), *Fruits of Solitude*. Retrieved from: http://www.bartleby.com/1/3/118.html

6. Thomas Jefferson, Letter to Maria Cosway, 1786. Retrieved from: http://www.pbs.org/jefferson/archives/documents/frame_ih195811.htm

CHAPTER 6

1. J. O. Prochaska, J. Norcross, and C. DiClemente, *Changing for Good* (New York: William Morrow Publishing, 1994).

2. Marshall B. Rosenberg, *Being Me, Loving You: A Practical Guide to Extraordinary Relationships* (Encinitas, CA: PuddleDancer Press, 2005).

CHAPTER 9

1. Alexander Pope (1688–1744), "The Universal Prayer" (poem). Retrieved from: http://www.poetryfoundation.org/poem/180945.

Create ♡ Morning Routine ♡
/Edit

1. Pour glass of H_2O drink
2. Feed Cats.
3. Pour another glass of H_2O
4. Pet Cats.
5. Put some pants on
   ☑ Stretch
       make som breakfast

| 1 egg + Egg (| Yogurt w/ Toppings |
| 1 egg (or white) | |
       Veggies /

Shower - Blow dry hair

Read Self care reform

Walk | / Cissy
              Chuck?
              Maura
Start Work ← Call

Print the things for
   cornell
   call Roofer
→ Pans for Carpet Clean ?

Made in the USA
Columbia, SC
25 June 2020